C   n

Eliz   .D.

Contemporary Books

Chicago New York San Francisco Lisbon London Madrid Mexico City
Milan New Delhi San Juan Seoul Singapore Sydney Toronto

Library of Congress Cataloging-in-Publication Data

Connell, Elizabeth B.
        The contraception sourcebook / Elizabeth B. Connell.
            p.   cm.
        Includes index.
        ISBN 0-7373-0403-0 (acid-free paper)
        1. Contraception.   2. Birth control.   3. Consumer education.
    I. Title.

    RG136.C535   2001
    613.9′4—dc21   2001042236

Contemporary Books

A Division of The McGraw-Hill Companies

1 2 3 4 5 6 7 8 9 0   DOC/DOC   0 9 8 7 6 5 4 3 2 1

ISBN 0-7373-0403-0

This book was set in Sabon
Printed and bound by R. R. Donnelley—Crawfordsville

Cover design by Anne LoCascio
Interior design by Rattray Design

McGraw-Hill books are available at special quantity discounts to use as premiums and sales promotions, or for use in corporate training programs. For more information, please write to the Director of Special Sales, Professional Publishing, McGraw-Hill, Two Penn Plaza, New York, NY 10121-2298. Or contact your local bookstore.

This book is printed on acid-free paper.

To Howard Tatum—colleague, friend, and husband
And to our nine children

Contents

FOREWORD ix

INTRODUCTION xi

1. THE HISTORY OF CONTRACEPTION 1

2. ORAL CONTRACEPTIVES 10
   History 10
   Pharmacology 13
   Types of Oral Contraceptives 15
   Mechanism of Action 17
   Over-the-Counter-Pill Use 18
   Efficacy 19
   Use of Oral Contraceptives 20
   Directions for Use 26
   Noncontraceptive Health Benefits 29
   Hormonal Effects of Oral Contraceptives 35
   Evaluation of Side Effects 55
   Assessment of Pill Side Effects 57
   Possible Adverse Side Effects of Oral Contraceptive Use 60
   Clinical Management of Side Effects 68
   Medical Considerations 73
   Return of Fertility 91
   Fetal Effects 92

Myths   93
Counseling   94
Resting   95
Compliance/Continuation   95
Progestin-Only Oral Contraceptives   97
Emergency Contraception   99
Future Trends   105
Summary   106

3. CONTRACEPTIVE IMPLANTS   107
Insertions   109
Removals   110
Side Effects   111
Advantages   111
Disadvantages   112
Continuation Rates   112
Candidates for Use   112
Counseling   113
Litigation   114
Future Implants   116

4. INJECTABLE CONTRACEPTIVES   118
Administration   122
Effectiveness   123
Advantages   123
Bleeding Patterns   125
Cultural Attitudes   126
Disadvantages   127
Cancer   128
Osteoporosis   129
Future Fertility   130
Fetal Effects   131
Contraindications   131
Usage   132
New Injectables   133

5. INTRAUTERINE DEVICES   136
History   136
Development   136

Current IUDs   138

Dalkon Shield   141

Mechanisms of Action   142

Effectiveness   144

Insertion   144

Side Effects/Complications   148

Advantages   155

Disadvantages   156

Good Candidates for IUD Use   156

Poor Candidates for IUD Use   157

Instructions for Use   158

Myths and Misperceptions   160

Usage   161

Future IUDs   164

6. FEMALE BARRIER CONTRACEPTIVES   166

Spermicides   168

Diaphragm   171

Cervical Cap   175

Vaginal Contraceptive Sponge   178

Female Condom   182

7. PERIODIC ABSTINENCE   185

Methods   186

Congenital Anomalies   188

Effectiveness   189

Advantages   190

Disadvantages   190

8. LACTATIONAL AMENORRHEA   192

Effectiveness   193

Contraceptive Options   194

9. ADDITIONAL METHODS OF FEMALE CONTRACEPTION   197

Vaginal Rings   197

Contraceptive Patches   198

Contraceptive Gels   199

Female Sterilization   199

Douching   203

Female Immunologic Methods   204

10.   MALE CONTRACEPTION   205
       Withdrawal   206
       Condoms   209
       Male Sterilization   213
       Medical Approaches   215
       Male Immunological Methods   218
       Male Reactions   218

11.   THE CURRENT STATUS OF CONTRACEPTION   220
       The Need for Better Contraception   220
       *The Current Status of Contraceptive Research and
          Development*   222
       Funding Sources   225
       Drug and Device Regulation   227
       Innovation Versus Liability   231
       Political Considerations   234
       The Doctor–Patient Relationship   235
       The Loss of the U.S. Leadership Role   237

12.   THE FUTURE OF CONTRACEPTION   238

       EPILOGUE   241

       SUGGESTED READING   243

       INDEX   249

Foreword

No one in America is better qualified to have written *The Contraception Sourcebook*. Dr. Elizabeth Connell, an internationally recognized scholar and teacher in contraception, knows her subject from many perspectives, reflecting her long, varied, and illustrious career. She has been a practitioner of obstetrics and gynecology in both private practice and academe. She has been a trusted advisor to the Food and Drug Administration. She helped to create the Standards and Guidelines for Planned Parenthood Federation of America. She has worked closely and effectively with both print and broadcast media over the years; I continue to enjoy seeing her featured on the television news, commenting on women's health issues.

As expected, this book is a gem. With her usual clear and engaging style, Dr. Connell tackles a broad range of topics in contraception. The introductory section on history gets the book off to a fun start. She continues to weave interesting historical highlights throughout the book—for example, in the section on coitus interruptus and its impact on the demographic transition. She makes a vast literature on contraceptive epidemiology easy to understand, avoiding the jargon that bogs down so many texts. She uses straightforward language, few numbers, and no boring tables—just narrative nuggets from the literature. The book is a blend of not only her comprehensive knowledge of the literature but also her years of experience caring for women. She knows the issues that concern women from a lifetime of clinical practice.

I anticipate that some readers will use this book as a text (to be read straight through) and others as a reference work, to look up specific questions: Does an important interaction exist between oral contraceptives and tetracycline? Do oral contraceptives influence the risk of breast cancer? Will the contraceptive sponge return to the U.S. market? How effective is tubal sterilization? *The Contraception Sourcebook* works well in both roles.

But beyond the pragmatic appeal of this book, readers will gain, especially in the final chapters, a sense of the visionary who wrote it. Elizabeth Connell's lifelong commitment to improving women's lives comes shining through these pages. As has been true all her life, she has the intellectual courage to say things that need to be said—and women everywhere will be the beneficiaries.

David A. Grimes, M.D.
Vice President of Biomedical Affairs
Family Health International
Research Triangle Park, North Carolina

Introduction

THERE IS NO more fascinating subject in medical history than the study of human fertility and the numerous attempts that have been made to control it. Over the centuries, people began to understand the steps involved in human reproduction and to search for ways to limit the number and to plan the timing of their children. The desired number of children has varied tremendously from one era to another, and from one culture to another, depending on individual situations and societal circumstances. Thus, in times of stress such as droughts or tribal migrations and, more recently, wars or financial depressions, birth rates have gone down. Conversely, when nations have been anxious to increase their power and military strength, birth rates have gone up. These trends have been well documented and actually occurred long before there were any means of safe and effective fertility control.

1

The History of Contraception

Over the course of human civilization, innumerable theories have developed with regard to the origins of pregnancy. As a result, a vast amount of fascinating folklore has evolved related to male and female roles. Many of these roles have been linked to certain animals and birds. At one time, it was believed that a woman became pregnant by bathing in a stream containing eels. It was also thought that a male child could enter its mother in the shape of a serpent; a female child could enter in the shape of a snail. Another interesting theory was that of the wandering womb child. This was reported to be a toad-shaped creature that crawled in and out of a woman's mouth while she was asleep. If it left in search of food and water and the woman shut her mouth while it was away, then the creature could not get back into the woman's mouth and consequently she would be childless. Albert the Great believed that if a woman spit three times into the mouth of a frog, she would be unable to conceive.

Many other beliefs were related to the spirit world in which the formation of babies had nothing to do with sexual intercourse. For example, Nordic folklore described a spirit child that lived in certain lakes and streams and in the fruits of certain trees. A woman who bathed in one of these bodies of water or who ate a fruit from one of the trees that contained a spirit child would become pregnant. Even today some Australian Aborigines believe that spirit children are responsible for the birth of babies.

The practice of wearing specific animal parts was thought to help women avoid unwanted pregnancy. For example, infertility could be induced by carrying a cat's liver in a tube on the left foot, tying the testicles of a cat at one's waist, or, even more effective, wearing the uterus of a lioness.

Certain birds were also believed to play a key role in fertility. For example, Hindus and Egyptians believed that the ibis was the bird that ensured a pregnancy; couples who were getting married and wanted many children offered up prayers to these birds when they saw flocks of them flying overhead. Other cultures attributed fertility to different species. The Japanese believed that pregnancy was related to the butterfly and the crane; Mexicans believed the red spoonbill was responsible. Several centuries ago, the ancient Teutons thought that storks brought babies. If they did not want any more children, they tried to drive the storks away. Since this did not seem to work, they concluded that storks brought babies mostly at night when they could not be seen. Interestingly, the visual image of an infant being carried by a stork still persists today.

The roles played by gender in the production of a pregnancy were explained in a variety of creative and interesting ways. One theory was that the entire baby came from the body of the mother and that all of its parts were formed in miniature in her abdomen prior to development and birth. Another belief was that the actual contribution to the pregnancy was exclusively that of the male—the role of the female was simply to nourish the baby until the time of its birth. Consequently, in wartime, captured males were put to death; women were kept as concubines since they contributed nothing to the development of a baby and therefore could not contaminate the heredity of the victors.

Perception of the role of the menses was also highly variable. Some cultures believed that a woman was always pregnant; therefore, any bleeding indicated that she had sustained an internal injury or had developed a serious disease. In other cultures, menstrual blood was perceived to be the way in which a woman's body rid itself of excess food; when her bleeding stopped with pregnancy, it was because the food was being diverted to feed the developing embryo. A Hindu theory held that the menstrual blood was the origin of the embryo. This led to the practice of child marriage, as the loss of menses prior to marriage was considered to represent the murder of babies.

History reports that Cleopatra ordered that her slaves be dissected to determine how the human body was constructed. Many centuries later, early anatomists robbed graves in pursuit of the same knowledge. As a result of these combined efforts, the various structures of the male and female reproductive tracts were gradually fairly well described. However, investigations into how they functioned—and particularly into how they could be controlled—were not carried out until much later. According to legend, Cleopatra reportedly had her slaves examined at the various stages of pregnancy to determine how their fetuses developed.

Once it was discovered, there was considerable interest in the uterus. Ancient Egyptians regarded it as an independent animal and believed that it could perform many types of movement. A uterus was also believed to have the ability to assume different forms—a crocodile, for example, or a tortoise. Hippocrates claimed that when a uterus was not fed with sufficient male sperm, it often went wild. In ancient times the Greeks felt that boys developed more quickly because they grew in the right side of the uterus which was warmer, whereas girls developed more slowly because they grew in the left side of the uterus, which was cooler.

The placenta also played a key role in the folklore of pregnancy. In Ancient Egypt, it was believed to be the center of life and the soul. Therefore, it was highly venerated. Pictures of placentas appear in some examples of the artwork of that period.

Methods for the prevention of unwanted pregnancy depended upon what theory of causation prevailed at the time. Once the actual contributions of the male and the female and the functions of the uterus and sperm came to be known, the same general approaches to contraception were used that we continue to see today. Medical history points out that virtually all the current methods of contraception had antecedents in earlier times. For example, once the association was made between the ejaculate and pregnancy, numerous exotic vaginal barriers were constructed by women to block the passage of sperm into the uterus. Moreover, both men and women have over the course of history swallowed an amazing array of concoctions (some of them lethal), the predecessors of the oral contraceptives. (Oral contraception will be discussed thoroughly in Chapter 2.)

One of the most fascinating elements in the history of contraception is the wide array of materials women have, over the years, placed in their vaginas to obstruct the passage of semen. One basic approach was to fashion pessaries from the excrement of powerful animals such as the elephant and the crocodile, held together by a paste made of honey, whitewash, or animal earwax. Some were made in the shape of a penis; others had a string attached to aid in removal. Many different types of plant and animal products were added to these pessaries, including the inner skin of a pomegranate, gallnut, and cabbage leaves.

In 1552 Spaniards reported that the Aztecs practiced contraception by placing the crushed herb of the calabash or cucurbita root and eagle excrement into a woman's vagina. They also recommended burning a lizard and mixing its ashes with wine and honey to make a pessary. Since the leaf of the sicklewort plant was sword-shaped, it was suggested that women coat it with honey and place it in their vaginas prior to intercourse. Also a hollowed-out half of a pomegranate was used as a cervical cap. A much more hazardous approach employed in Central Africa was to chop grass and linen into fine pieces and use them to plug up the vagina; this practice often caused severe complications and frequently death because the plugs blocked the passage of urine and feces.

A few of these pessaries actually had some biologic plausibility. For example, a half of a lemon, being highly acidic, placed over the cervix might well have had some degree of effectiveness. It was also found that some plants that were used in Sumatra for this purpose had high levels of tannic acid, which is known to be spermicidal. Another approach was taken in Persia in the tenth century; rock salt, also spermicidal, was mixed with an oily material to make pessaries. At about the same time in Baghdad, the physician and scholar Avicenna recommended mixing alum, an efficient spermicide, with the pulp of a pomegranate. The resulting pessary also caused contraction of the vagina, a phenomenon that was considered desirable after vaginal stretching due to childbirth. In addition, Avicenna advised women to dip wool in the juice of the weeping willow and insert it into the vagina before coitus and to install pepper afterward. A slightly more bizarre method was to insert a wolf testicle that had been rubbed with oil and wool prior to sexual intercourse.

Other materials used as barriers included sponges taken from the ocean and wads of feathers. Oiled silk paper called *misugami* was used in China and Japan; it was rolled up into a ball and placed in the vagina. Slovak women, on the other hand, used clean linen rags. In Hungary, women reportedly melted beeswax and molded it into discs, which they then placed in their vaginas before intercourse.

Men also developed their own forms of contraception. Condoms, also known as sheaths, were used in ancient times; they appear in prehistoric cave drawings. Some of the first condoms were made out of animal intestines and bladders. Other materials reportedly were used in Asia. The Chinese fashioned sheaths of oiled silk paper. The Japanese invented the *Kabuta-Gata*, a device made of tortoiseshell or leather that was used to block the ejaculate; it was reportedly also of help to impotent men.

It was reported that Casanova had gold made into eighteen millimeter balls that he inserted into the vaginas of his numerous lady friends to prevent them from becoming pregnant. He stated that each one could be used for at least fifteen years. Casanova also used condoms, which he termed "English Riding Coats." However, he did not particularly like them because they "felt like a piece of dead skin."

Another type of contraceptive approach that was used just prior to intercourse involved a special kettle with a long thin spout on top, for women to sit on. Live coals sprinkled with neem wood were placed in the kettle; the steam which was generated went through the spout into the vagina and acted as a spermicide. After intercourse, douching with substances such as wine and garlic mixed with fennel was advised. The douches were administered using several different types of devices—the bill of the ibis, tubes made of wood and ivory, and lead pipes with a sponge at one end.

Some cultures believed that physically ridding the vagina of semen could prevent pregnancy. Women coughed, sneezed, or jumped to force the semen out of the vagina after ejaculation. Avicenna recommended taking seven jumps backward after intercourse, sneezing at the same time (it was important to jump backward because jumping forward would not dislodge the sperm). Running and dancing were other ways by which it was believed that a woman could expel the ejaculate.

Three major contraceptive techniques to be employed at the time of coitus have been described. One did not work and was soon discarded; one reportedly reduced pregnancy rates by 80 percent; and one very ancient method is still widely used today. The first was called *coitus saxonicus* and was practiced in the early fourteenth century. Just prior to ejaculation, the woman pressed hard on the base of the penis, attempting to force the ejaculate up into the bladder. The second was known as *coitus reservatus*, also called *Karezza* or male continence. In this instance, a man did not ejaculate during intercourse; he allowed his erection to subside while his penis was still inside the vagina. This method was endorsed by the utopian Oneida Community, which was founded by John Noyes in New York in 1847 and was reported to eliminate "the old idea of man's domination over women." The third method was called *coitus interruptus*, or withdrawal, with ejaculation taking place outside the vagina. This well-known practice was described in the Old Testament Book of Genesis 38, when Onan "spilled the seed on the ground lest he should give seed to his brother" when he was ordered by his father Judah to have intercourse with the wife of his dead brother, Er.

There have also been a number of emotional approaches recommended over the centuries to prevent unwanted pregnancies. In 1100 B.C. the Chinese called an example of this type of birth control *Kong Fou*. "At the moment of ejaculation," the advice went, "draw a deep breath and think of other things." Unfortunately history does not relate what sorts of "things" were most effective. In 1700 Musitanus claimed that women should avoid passionate intercourse if they did not want to become pregnant. In a number of cultures, it was believed that the enjoyment of coitus was satanical and would result in unwanted babies.

For centuries women have taken a wide variety of preparations orally in order to avoid or terminate pregnancy. One of the first primitive oral contraceptives (OC) described was silphium, a plant used in the fourth century B.C. It proved extremely effective—and therefore popular—and the plant became extinct by the third or fourth century A.D. Most of the earliest oral preparations were made from the bark of trees such as poplar and pine, and from dozens of different plants, including pineapple, asparagus, cabbage, onion, milkweed, thistle, sage, rosemary, and ivy. More than two thousand years ago, Hippocrates recommended the use of Queen Anne's lace as an oral contraceptive. The seeds of the castor oil plant were widely used in Europe and the Middle East.

Parts of animals were also employed as birth control methods often taken, not surprisingly, from male genitalia. One concoction used a wolf penis boiled in water; another recipe suggested taking the same organ from a bull, then drying it and making it into a powder to be added to soup. The well-known "Moroccan revenge" was bread containing hoof parings from a mule. Since the mule was sterile, it was believed that eating this food would render women permanently unable to have a child

In the Middle Ages, many women became ill and some died when they ingested mercury, arsenic, lead, iron, copper, iodine, and strychnine in their attempts to either prevent or end unwanted pregnancies. In the 1800s, Canadian women developed a contraceptive preparation by boiling dried beaver testicles in alcohol.

Use of the chastity belt, "the girdle of chastity," often made of gold or copper and fashioned in fanciful forms such as winged monsters and griffins—the traditional guardians of treasures—is well documented. In Biblical times they were called *Koomuz*; the name was derived from Kahn, Mokolm, and Zimo (KMZ), a place of extramarital sexual intercourse. Chastity belts covered most of the vulva and sometimes the anus and had two small holes to allow the passage of urine and menses. To prevent adultery and the birth of illegitimate children, men locked these contraptions onto their wives before going off to the Crusades. A variation on the belt design was a ring that held the labia together.

Somewhat less well known is the male practice of infibulation, the insertion of a ring or clasp through the foreskin of the penis to prevent intercourse. These devices were reportedly applied to Roman soldiers before they left for war. A somewhat less effective method was advocated by Pliny the Elder: "Rub crushed juniper berries all over the male part before coition to prevent conception."

There are many references in ancient literature to procedures designed to sterilize individuals of both sexes. Removal of the ovaries was practiced by the ancient Egyptians. Certain Australian tribes castrated boys before the age of puberty as a means of population control in times of famine. Both men and women subjected themselves to extensive, frequently mutilating, and sometimes lethal surgical procedures to control fertility. A procedure known as *Koolpi* was practiced on men in primitive Australia. The urethra was slit in front of the scrotum and, in even more extreme procedures, the entire urethra was laid open.

Equally drastic measures were performed on the female. A procedure called *Eurilthas* involved placing emu feathers in the vagina and uterus for several days. They were then removed along with part of the uterus, and the vaginal opening was opened as far back as the anus. Another diabolic practice described in medical history was the forcible jumping up and down on the abdomen of a woman in order to produce an abortion or to destroy her capacity to bear children. Finally, abortion has always been widely practiced over the centuries, not only by the oral use of herbs and other chemical agents, but also by the direct invasion of the pregnant uterus with a variety of instruments and abortifacients. These measures often proved fatal, due to hemorrhage and infection.

Fortunately, all of these practices were gradually superseded by far safer and more effective birth control measures, aided in large part by the discovery of the presence of sperm in seminal fluid in 1677 by Antonie van Leeuwenhoek, a Dutch naturalist. Once this discovery had been made, modern methods of contraception began to be developed based on science rather than on the fascinating but often unscientific theories that had been operative up until that time.

Thus, despite the tremendous interest that people have always shown in the control of their fertility, truly scientific research into this very important area is of fairly recent origin. Only in the twentieth century did contraceptive development move into an era that resulted in a number of techniques that actually were both safe and effective.

The objective at that time was (and continues to be) to find the "ideal contraceptive," one that is totally safe, totally effective, highly acceptable, inexpensive, readily reversible, easy to administer, easy to transport and store, and can be used at a time unrelated to sexual intercourse. Another perquisite, added more recently to the definition, is one that can help to protect against the transmission of sexually transmitted diseases (STDs).

2

Oral Contraceptives

History

IN THE 1920S, when female hormones were first studied, two scientists in Austria, Ludwig Haberlandt and Otfried Otto Fellner, began to think that they might be useful as a form of birth control. They based their hypothesis on the fact that when extracts made of these steroids were given to animals, their fertility could be inhibited. However, obtaining sufficient materials for research in the human female posed a serious problem. For example, it took 80,000 sow ovaries to produce just 12 mg of an estrogen known as estradiol. Moreover, it took the ovaries from 2,500 pregnant pigs to produce 1 mg of progesterone.

An outstanding pioneer who began to work in this field was an American, Russell E. Marker. He concluded that the only way to get large quantities of steroid hormones was to find plants that made a steroid called diosgenin. In 1942, after searching in Mexico for several years, Marker finally found one that contained this material; it was the Mexican yam. After tremendous difficulties and with virtually no financial support (he had to exhaust his life's savings), he eventually worked out a technique whereby one gallon of syrup taken from the roots of the yam would yield 3 kilograms of progesterone. Returning to Mexico in 1943, he collected ten tons of yams, and, along with two Mexicans—one a lawyer and one a physician—formed a company

(Syntex), which then began to produce progesterone, marketed at $200 a gram.

Another key figure was Carl Djerassi, the son of two Bulgarian physicians. After emigrating to the United States in 1939 and being trained in chemistry, he began to work at Syntex, attempting to synthesize cortisone for the treatment of arthritis. When progesterone was found to be an excellent base material in the manufacture of cortisone, Syntex began to produce ten tons a year, selling it at forty-eight cents per gram. The first orally active progestational agent—norethynodrel—was developed by Frank Colton at G. D. Searle & Company. Then in 1951, Djerassi and others at Syntex developed another of the first progestins—norethindrone—that could be taken by mouth.

A third key player in this development was Gregory Goodwin Pincus, a brilliant biologist with a strong dedication to the development of products that would be useful in solving some of the major problems faced by human beings, particularly those posed by the rapidly expanding world population. He was joined in this work at Clark University by Hudson Hoagland, and then by Min-Chueh Chang. They, like their predecessor Marker, not only received very little support but also got considerable antagonism from the scientific community. However, by raising money from private sources, they were able to continue their research. This ultimately led to the 1945 establishment of an institution now world-renowned, known as the Worcester Foundation for Experimental Biology.

In 1951, Chang showed that both norethynodrel and norethindrone, when administered orally to rabbits, consistently blocked ovulation. At that point the search for products to use in the human female began in earnest.

In the same year, an important meeting occurred, one that was to have a major impact on the development and use of the oral contraceptives. Pincus visited with Margaret Sanger, honorary president of the Planned Parenthood Federation of America and an outstanding leader in the field of birth control for women. One of the best-known and most often repeated episodes in contraceptive history was the time when Margaret Sanger told a poor woman who had already had more babies than she wanted or could support that her only solution was to tell her husband, Jake, to go and sleep on the roof of their New York tenement. It also was at about the same time that Eleanor Roosevelt, after the birth of her sixth child, announced to her husband, Franklin, that their sexual life together was over; she could not face another pregnancy and yet was powerless to prevent it. Margaret Sanger encouraged Pincus and Chang to pursue their laboratory studies to find products that could be made, distributed widely, and used safely and effectively by women.

Another woman, key to this entire effort, was Kathryn Dexter McCormick. She was an extremely wealthy woman married to the son of Cyrus McCormick, the head of International Harvester. She was only the second woman to graduate from the Massachusetts Institute of Technology (MIT). Like Margaret Sanger, she was also deeply dedicated to the health-care field, particularly family planning. In 1952, Pincus arranged to meet with both Sanger and McCormick. They were greatly impressed by his research and became highly supportive. They provided money for further animal studies; ultimately McCormick gave more than $2 million to the Worchester Foundation and left it an additional $1 million in her will.

At about this time Pincus recognized that he needed to have a physician who would work with him in the future development of contraceptive products for use by women. He fortuitously met Dr. John Rock, a well-known researcher, who was then the head of gynecology at Harvard. They began to collaborate and did outstanding research determining the details of the fertilization of human eggs in the laboratory, in 1944 reporting the first in-vitro fertilization. Interestingly, when they first met, Rock was studying the same progestational agents as Pincus; he was hoping that they would be of value in his work on infertility. Once it was recognized that they in fact produced infertility by blocking ovulation, they worked together to produce the first oral contraceptives (OCs). It has been reported that Sanger and McCormick were originally very concerned about working with Dr. Rock, despite his outstanding scientific credentials, because he was a practicing Roman Catholic. However, his great dedication to solving population problems was apparent, and they gradually became extremely supportive. The first clinical trials were carried out in 1954 on fifty of Rock's patients by Dr. Luigi Mastroianni; none of them ovulated.

These hormones were studied further in the human female in 1956 by Doctors Celso-Ramon Garcia and Edris Rice-Wray, working in Puerto Rico. Following this, additional clinical trials were conducted by Dr. Joseph W. Goldzieher in San Antonio, Texas, and Dr. Edward T. Tyler in Los Angeles, California.

When all of these trials began to look very promising, G. D. Searle & Company became interested in the manufacture and sale of an oral contraceptive. Following additional research, in 1960 Searle obtained FDA approval for marketing a pill for contraception named Enovid; it contained 150 mcg of mestranol and 9.85 mg of norethynodrel. Two other pharmaceutical companies, Ortho in 1962 and Wyeth Laboratories in 1968, also began to produce and market their own versions of "the Pill," as it was originally called by Pincus.

The introduction of the pill coincided with (and undoubtedly played a major role in) the era of women's liberation, a time during which women began to demand reproductive freedom and control over their own bodies. It also occurred at a time when women were beginning to achieve higher levels of education and thus could look forward to more creative and productive careers. Now, for the first time in their lives, sexually active women could be freed from their anxiety about having an unwanted pregnancy, and consequently could begin to plan their lives. Of great interest in this regard is a comment made by Pincus in 1957. "How a few precious facts obscurely come in to the laboratory may resonate into the lives of men everywhere, bring order to disorders, hope to the hopeless, life to the dying." When he himself died in 1967, he along with many others had been responsible for one of the few precious facts.

Pharmacology

Estrogen

The earlier oral contraceptives contained two hormones, one of which was an estrogen, either mestranol or ethinyl estradiol. Some animal studies suggested that mestranol was weaker, and therefore it was gradually formulated out of the OCs. Almost all of the low-dose preparations available today contain ethinyl estradiol.

Progestins

The currently available OCs contain a variety of different progestational agents. These include the earlier so-called first generation progestins such as norethindrone and norethynodrel and the second-generation progestins such as levonorgestrel and norgestimate.

A major controversy erupted in October 1995 when the United Kingdom's (UK) Committee on the Safety of Medicine (CSM) leaked information to the press, before telling the British doctors, that the so-called third generation of progestins—desogestrel and gestodene—posed twice the risk of venous thromboembolism (VTE) as compared with the earlier progestins. This conclusion was drawn from several large unpublished studies, primarily one from the World Health Organization (WHO). As one would have predicted, this announcement set off a "pill scare," resulting in panic among women; OC use dropped sharply and, predictably, there was also an increase in unwanted pregnancies and in elective induced abortions. The British doctors were also very upset because they were unaware of the studies inasmuch as none of the data had ever been published, and they were unsure about how to respond to the many questions posed by their anxious patients. It was subsequently suggested by a number of investigators, both in the United Kingdom and elsewhere, after reviewing the reports, that there was considerable bias in the studies, a fact that rendered them of questionable significance. Many health-care professionals also felt that the CSM had badly overreacted and created an unnecessary situation.

The bottom line of the controversy (which still continues) is that there is not sufficient evidence to regard the third-generation progestins as having risks that would justify discontinuing their use. A November 24, 1995, FDA report stated that the risks were not great enough to recommend switching to other OCs. The American College of Obstetricians and Gynecologists (ACOG) backed this position about a year later. However, the manufacturers of one of the desogestrel-containing pills did add language in the warning section of their package insert, detailing the findings of the studies regarding VTE risk.

To put this matter into proper perspective, it is important to recognize that the risk of thromboembolism in pregnancy was at least two times that found with the studies on these agents. Moreover, clinicians were reminded that to help to avoid this complication, it was always necessary to take a careful history looking for risk factors for VTEs such as prior thromboembolic events; a family history of this condition; and other factors such as obesity, immobilization, and recent surgery.

Recent research has found no evidence for a two-fold increase in the risk of thromboembolism with the third-generation progestins.

Potency

The effectiveness of any oral contraceptive depends upon the potency of the hormone or hormones that it contains. Potency is measured by both animal and human testing. Many different types of evaluations have been used in animals, looking at changes in certain body tissues and the impacts of OCs on pregnancies. A commonly used test in women is the delay of menses which occurs when the product is being administered.

However, it is well recognized that animal data may not be directly transferred to the human, nor is it possible to determine the potency of a combined oral contraceptive by measuring the potency of the estrogen and the progestin separately, and then attempting to combine them. The measured potency of any drug varies widely depending on the species being tested, the route of administration, and the tissues being analyzed. Therefore, it is impossible to look at a single test in either an animal or a human and use it as a definitive test for the potency of a particular drug. Too often this has been done, leading to claims that are good for sales but are without adequate clinical evidence.

Types of Oral Contraceptives

The oral contraceptives that we are using today are dramatically different from the first one approved in 1960. Over time, it was recognized that the amounts of the two hormones put in the earlier contraceptives to ensure that ovulation was suppressed were far in excess of what was actually required. The dosages of both hormones were dropped progressively over a period of many years; the original pill had four times as much estrogen and almost ten times as much progestin as the current preparations. These changes led to a decrease in the adverse side effects that women were noticing; however, it had no impact on the high level of efficacy found with the earlier pills.

There are close to fifty different OC preparations made in the United States and other countries today. They fall into two basic types: the combined pill, which contains both an estrogen and a progestin, and the minipill, which has a progestin only. The first type of combination pill that was made was monophasic in character, that is, the estrogen and the progestin were given throughout the entire twenty-one-day pill cycle in a constant dosage. Following this, the medication was stopped and for the next week no pills were taken. Somewhat later, a placebo such as sugar pills (or in the case of some developing countries, iron tablets) was administered instead of stopping for a week. The change to the second approach occurred because women found it easier to remember to take their pills properly if they took one tablet every day. After this OC-free week, the tablets containing the active ingredients were restarted. Pills packaged this way were known as "memory packets." Almost all of the combined pills available today, regardless of type, are made in either twenty-one-day or twenty-eight-day cycles.

Somewhat later, the sequential pill was developed, based on the assumption that hormones given in this fashion were more similar to the pattern of the normal untreated menstrual cycle. The estrogen was given alone for about two weeks, a progestin was added to the same dose of estrogen for another week, and then both were discontinued for seven days. After several years of use of these OCs, one of the sequential preparations was reported to increase the risk of endometrial cancer. Therefore, it was disapproved by the FDA. The other sequential preparations were also voluntarily discontinued, although there was no evidence at that time that they had a similar problem.

Next, the phasic pills were developed. The first type was the biphasic OC. In this formulation, the estrogen and progestin doses remained constant for about two weeks, the progestin dose was increased for the last week of treatment, and then a placebo was given for seven days. Next, the triphasic OCs were developed. Here again the estrogen dosage remained constant but the progestin dose varied in each of three phases, different pills having different dosage patterns. Phasic pills, like the sequentials, were claimed to be more physiologic, being similar in design to the normal menstrual cycle. However, since the hormones had to be given in pharmacological not physiologic doses to be effective, this claim was not really scientifically valid.

Over the years, questions continued to be raised about the safety of the higher dose pills, particularly the potential for thromboembolic complications due to the estrogen. In 1993, the FDA informed the pharmaceutical companies making oral contraceptives that dosages over 50 mcg of estrogen should be voluntarily removed from the market. At a meeting of the FDA's advisory panel, it was suggested that even the 50 mcg pills should possibly be discontinued. However, it was pointed out that, in certain instances, there was a clear need for these pills. This was particularly true when bleeding problems occurred with lower-dose pills. There were also certain medical indications for the use of the 50 mcg oral contraceptives, such as situations where drug-interaction studies had suggested that the lower-dose pills would be less effective. The majority of the committee members recommended leaving the 50 mcg estrogen-containing OCs on the market; however, the committee stressed that labeling should emphasize that prescriptions should contain the smallest estrogen dose necessary for contraceptive effectiveness.

Mechanism of Action

All of the combined oral contraceptives, regardless of subtype, produce their effects by blocking ovulation. The hormones in the OCs act on the parts of the brain that control the development and expulsion of eggs from the ovaries, and over time the ovaries gradually decrease in size. Another change is seen in the endometrium, the lining of the uterine cavity; it becomes progressively thinner and less active. In addition, because of the progestin, changes occur in the endocervical mucus which block the passage of sperm from the vagina up into the uterine cavity. It has also been suggested but never proved that the hormones alter, in some way, the functions of the fallopian tubes.

Over-the-Counter-Pill Use

In many countries, oral contraceptives have been made available outside the traditional health-care systems. They have been dispensed by pharmacies, clinics, and a variety of community-distribution programs, allowing use of the OCs where they had previously been unavailable. In some areas, this approach has worked extremely well; in others it has not proved particularly useful.

In the mid-1970s, Sweden passed a law that allowed women to have free and legal abortions prior to the eighteenth week of pregnancy. At that time there was considerable concern that many women might rely on abortion rather than use contraception so, in an attempt to prevent this, pills were made available over-the-counter (OTC). However, this approach turned out to be not as successful as had been hoped. Confusion about how to take the drugs resulted in poor pill-taking and confirmed the fact that counseling is exceedingly important and may, in fact, be absolutely critical to good compliance and continuation. In the teenage group, it was found that girls were using each other's pills and that missed pills and irregular bleeding were commonplace. Many of them stopped using the pill because they felt that taking it was too much trouble. As time went on, surveys showed that the sales of the oral contraceptives had actually dropped. In response to this situation, Sweden set up training programs for nurse-midwives. At present about 80 percent of Sweden's OCs are prescribed by these individuals. Compliance rates have improved, and Sweden now has significantly lower teenage-pregnancy and abortion rates than the United States.

Multiple attempts have been made to assess whether or not OCs should be made available OTC in the United States. Two different (and often confrontational) schools of thought have emerged. Those in favor feel that doing so would increase access to contraception for those who do not want to become involved, for one reason or another, in the traditional health-care system. They believe that many women, particularly teenagers, who do not want to have blood drawn and have pelvic examinations performed would see this as a way of preventing unwanted pregnancy without having to go through the usual forms of medical care. Other arguments made in favor of having pills available OTC include increased availability and confidentiality, less time spent trying to get into the health-care system and less administrative cost.

On the other side is the long-standing concern, now reinforced by the Swedish experience, that without good counseling, there will be poor compliance and continuation. Another major objection is that without adequate screening, even with good labeling, women who should not use OCs might do so. Opponents to making the oral contraceptives available OTC cite a number of reasons for women to get their pills by prescription. These include getting breast exams and learning the technique of breast self-examination, access to smoking-cessation programs and dietary counseling, training in the proper use of the pill, and the availability of medical guidance in the event that there are problems. Also physical and pelvic examinations might pick up medical conditions that would otherwise go unnoticed such as STDs and early cervical cancers. Another concern is that blood pressures would not be checked. While this is not critical very often in the younger age group, it becomes much more so as women get older.

Thus the debate continues in the United States. The overall risk/benefit ratio of allowing open access to OCs remains unresolved and is a highly volatile issue from ethical, financial, and public-health points of view. In general, the low-dose pills are felt to be safe and effective for the vast majority of women. In addition, noncontraceptive health benefits of OCs are proving increasingly significant; many medical practitioners believe that as many women as possible should receive these protections. In fact, some have suggested that even women who do not need protection against unwanted pregnancies should take OCs for several years in order to get related health benefits.

Efficacy

The OCs are among the most effective forms of birth control ever developed. Women using these preparations properly have a nearly

100 percent rate of protection. However, studies have shown that when pills are not taken according to instructions—unfortunately very often the case—the failure rates rise to between 3 and 6 percent and often even higher. Furthermore, these levels of effectiveness have remained constant despite the progressive lowering of the amounts of both estrogen and progestin in the pills.

Most of the failures reported with OC use have been due to missed pills. Failures have also been found to be age-related; pregnancies are more common in younger women and become progressively less common as women grow older. It is very important that women understand that there are major differences in the effectiveness of OCs depending on how well they are taken. It repeatedly has been shown that women usually tend to think of the effectiveness of the pill in terms of the rates reported with perfect use.

Use of Oral Contraceptives

Issues Related to Age

For a long time there was considerable debate about whether it was appropriate to use OCs at the beginning and at the end of a woman's reproductive life.

First, there was consternation as to whether or not use of the pill in a girl just passing through puberty would stunt her growth. This fear was eventually put to rest by the delayed recognition that as part of a young girl's normal development, her largest growth spurt occurs prior to her menarche. By the time she begins to ovulate and have menstrual periods, her epiphyses (areas of bone growth) are already virtually closed, and therefore there is no reason to believe that her ultimate height would be endangered by OC use. In fact, treatments using very large doses of estrogen in attempts to limit the ultimate height of some young girls were generally unsuccessful.

Another concern arose when young girls who had irregular menses were given the oral contraceptives, following which their periods became "normal." Then, upon stopping the OCs, they often again developed irregular periods, sometimes had episodes of amenorrhea, and often had difficulty becoming pregnant. Ultimately it became clear that the regular bleeding that occurred during the use of the OCs did not represent an improvement in gynecologic health; rather, in this case, it was secondary to the use of the OCs. Once the girls stopped taking the pill, they simply reverted to their previous gynecologic status. Thus this menstrual pattern did not represent a negative effect of the OCs on their reproductive potential. Therefore, there is no reason not to use oral contraceptives in this particular group; they may well go on to ovulate at some time and become pregnant. However, if there continues to be a problem, they need to have a careful medical evaluation, as would probably have been necessary in any event.

Second, there were concerns for many years about the use of the oral contraceptives in women over the age of thirty-five. In the era of the high-dose pills, these concerns were founded on the possible induction of cardiovascular disease; many felt it was inappropriate for women thirty-five years of age and older to take OCs. For a considerable period of time, labeling on the pills indicated that smokers should stop using the pill at age thirty-five and nonsmokers at forty. Then, as more research was carried out looking at the issue of OC use in the older age group, it became apparent that this guideline had led to an unnecessary curtailment of the use of oral contraceptives by many women over forty who were healthy, who did not smoke, and who wished to continue to take them. As the OC studies continued, it was eventually recognized that two factors—age and smoking—had their own particular cardiovascular risks. However, adding the two risks together did not indicate the true real risk; OC use plus smoking led to a total risk considerably greater than the sum of the two individual figures (synergism). Therefore current labeling quite appropriately still recommends discontinuation of OC use at age thirty-five if a woman is going to continue to smoke, particularly if she smokes heavily. However, there is no reason that healthy, nonsmoking women should not continue to take the pill as long as they so desire, even up to the time of their menopause. Moreover, although smoking carries an increased risk for younger women, it is not sufficiently large to deny them the use of OCs.

There are many good reasons to allow older women to use this highly effective form of birth control. The majority of pregnancies in women over age forty have been found to be unplanned and unwanted. For many years the number of elective abortions in the forty- to forty-four-year-old age group is second only to that of teenagers under the age of fifteen. Moreover, both maternal and infant morbidity and mortality rates become significantly higher as women grow older, as does the chance of having babies with congenital abnormalities and Down's syndrome.

Despite the increase in knowledge and the change in OC labeling, older women have been reluctant to use oral contraceptives; some health-care providers have unfortunately been equally slow in encouraging this age group to use the OCs. At the present time, there is an inverse ratio between pill use and age. Younger women use the pill about 70 to 80 percent of the time. However, the number of older women selecting this method of contraception declines sharply; most studies show that by the mid-forties, OC use declines to only about 3 to 5 percent.

Clinical Evaluation

Prior to selecting and beginning use of the pill, women should provide their health-care providers with detailed medical and family histories. Traditionally, this is followed by a thorough physical examination including a pelvic exam and a Papanicolaou smear as well as vaginal cultures, when indicated, and drawing of blood for laboratory testing. As noted elsewhere, there has recently been a major debate as to whether or not it is appropriate to temporarily defer the pelvic examination until after a patient has begun her oral birth control. Some clinicians now feel that taking a history, performing one of the new highly sensitive pregnancy tests if necessary, and measuring blood pressure is sufficient in this situation. The major disadvantage of this approach is that a sexually transmitted disease may be missed. However, the presence of an STD is not a contraindication to the use of oral contraceptives.

Several organizations have suggested that healthy young women should be allowed to defer these examinations and be given the oral contraceptives for two to three months, if this seems to be the most appropriate course. This approach will purportedly increase OC usage; the hope is that at the time of their follow-up pill resupply visit, these individuals will have established sufficient rapport with their clinicians for the deferred pelvic exam to be carried out, and thereafter will seek and receive standard health care.

Laboratory Testing

Over the years, there has been considerable discussion about whether or not all women needed to undergo certain laboratory tests prior to starting the oral contraceptives, or whether this should depend on their medical history and physical findings. Fairly extensive testing was originally recommended for all women, with a particular focus on lipid and glucose levels. However, with the advent of the low-dose pills that have minimal effects on metabolic changes, it is currently recommended that these be done only once, if at all, for healthy young women. Extensive and repeated laboratory testing ultimately was not found to be useful in the vast majority of instances, and was also extremely expensive. However, older women and those with risk factors such as diabetes, marked obesity, and those with a family history of diabetes and cardiovascular disease should be tested and reevaluated on a yearly basis.

Choice of an Oral Contraceptive

The pill of choice is one which offers a woman high levels of effectiveness and safety and has side effects that are generally acceptable. This usually means an estrogen dose of less than 50 mcg, and a progestin dose of less than 1 mg. There are two situations in which selection of a higher dose (50 mcg) pill may be appropriate. The first is in situations where there may be a drug interaction. The second is in the case of a woman who has excessively heavy menstrual periods. The monophasic higher-dose pills are usually more effective in helping with this problem than the multiphasic pills. Once the bleeding decreases, it is often possible to switch to a low-dose preparation.

Some of the multiphasic pills have less total progestin than some of the monophasic products. However, there appears to be no significant clinical difference between these two types and thus it is not a key selection factor in most cases. Women who started their oral contraceptive therapy in the era of higher dose pills should be switched to lower-dose preparations. This can usually be done without inducing an increased number of side effects, particularly abnormal bleeding. Also, it can be accomplished without any decrease in the level of effectiveness.

The potency of the hormones in the oral contraceptives, particularly the progestins, was a major consideration at one time. However, this is no longer an issue because the doses of both hormones have been adjusted in the existing pills based on studies of their own individual potencies. At one time, it was suggested that the choice of the proper pill can be tailor-made to fit each particular woman, depending on certain physical characteristics. However, there are no valid research data to suggest that this is a practical or even a feasible approach. In general, it is impossible to predict in advance exactly what the best pill might be for any individual woman. However, when the level of effectiveness is a matter of great concern, the choice of a combined pill over that of a minipill is preferable.

Pill Labeling

Every OC has a patient package insert, approved by the FDA, which is essentially the same for all pills. Manufacturers of the oral contraceptives are required to include an insert with each pill package. With the passage of time, these labels have gotten more and more detailed and, from a consumer perspective, less and less valuable. Unfortunately, they are now very lengthy, often quite technical and printed in extremely small letters. A number of the risks that are mentioned apply primarily to the higher-dose pills. Also the overall risk/benefit ratio is not well presented, which would be of great value to potential users.

As new information has come along, there have been periodic updates to OC labeling, incorporating the new scientific evidence. However, the FDA noted that a number of claims were being made that were not backed up by significant clinical data. Therefore, in 1991, it informed the OC manufacturers that they could not include in labeling anything without scientific validation and that they could not put any material in the patient package insert that was inherently promotional.

In 1993, the FDA advisory committee held hearings to try to obtain suggestions as to how to rewrite OC labeling to make it more understandable and useful to consumers. A number of people made suggestions as to how to simplify and restructure the labeling. The committee recommended a streamlined one-page summary of the labeling and a toll-free hotline for OC users. It was pointed out by a number of people at that meeting that the language in the labeling was far too complex for the average woman and that the current labeling often reflected data from the older high-dose pills which were no longer relevant to the newer low-dose pills.

A considerable delay has often occurred in the updating of information in the labeling, and claims that are no longer relevant serve only to confuse women and often produce fear, failure to start OC use, and discontinuations—to say nothing of an increased number of lawsuits. In 1993, additional labeling requirements were laid out by the FDA. Manufacturers of the oral contraceptives were told that they needed to include in their labeling the fact that their products were intended to prevent pregnancy but that they did not protect against transmission of HIV/AIDS or other STDs.

Usage

Ever since their introduction, OCs have been used all over the world. Today, in many countries, they remain the method of choice despite the introduction of newer methods. Current estimates claim that more than 100 million women rely on OCs to prevent unwanted pregnancy. Worldwide data show that 8 percent of all married women are now taking the pill; it ranks third, after female sterilization and the IUD. Worldwide usage is even higher among sexually active unmarried women; 26 percent of this group rely upon the oral contraceptives.

A survey carried out in sixty-eight developing countries showed that between 40 and 50 percent of married women selected the pill. In Latin America, 55 percent of all married women have used the pill, and in Brazil nearly 80 percent of married women have taken an OC at some point. Surveys of unmarried sexually active women show a similar pattern. In this group, the pill has been chosen more often than any other form of modern contraception. About 50 percent of all women surveyed had used OCs at some point.

In developed countries, the pill is the most used form of birth control; some 16 percent of married women choose the pill. (The condom and the IUD are the next most popular methods; both are used by 14 percent of married women.) Surveys provide much of these data. One from Canada in 1995 showed that 86 percent of women had used the pill, in the United States more than 80 percent, and in Germany—the highest use—94 percent of East German women between the ages of thirty and forty-four had used OCs. Other studies have reported that a large percentage of sexually active unmarried women in developed countries use the pill—36 percent in North America, and 45 percent in Europe.

There are major differences in the utilization of OCs depending on the area of the world being surveyed. The availability of the pill often depends upon the amount of support and involvement of both public and private organizations. The use of OCs is very limited in India and China. Japan has the lowest rate, less than 1 percent, since for a variety of reasons (primarily hypothetical) the OCs were only approved for the first time in September 1999.

Directions for Use

Starting OCs

In recent years, changes have also been made in the way women are told to start their oral contraceptives. As previously noted in the section on types of OCs, women used to count up to the fifth day of menstruation, start the pills, and then take them for twenty-one days. Then they either took no pills or a placebo for seven days and started again. They started the progestin-only pills on day one of a menstrual period and continued to take them daily.

More recently a different approach has gained popularity. This is called the "Sunday start." A woman will begin taking her medication if her menstrual period starts on a Sunday, but if it starts on any other day, she will wait until the following Sunday to begin her medication. However, for the combined pills, no more than six days should go by without starting a packet. In the case of the multiphasic oral contraceptives, many doctors advise that they be started on the first day of the menstrual period. This is because there is a lower dose of steroid in this type of preparation; consequently it is important to begin earlier to block ovulation in the first cycle. The Sunday start has been used increasingly because it is easy to remember and because it avoids the nuisance of withdrawal bleeding on weekends.

To ensure sufficient protection, some doctors suggest that all their patients use a barrier contraceptive during the first week. The usual pattern of OC use may be changed if desired for a special reason. For example, if a woman wishes to postpone having her menstrual period because of a special occasion such as a wedding or a vacation, she may omit the seven days when no active pill is taken and immediately start a new pack, beginning with the hormone-bearing pills.

A woman who has delivered a full-term baby is advised that the pill start be delayed for two weeks because of the very small risk of a venous thrombosis. However, with low-dose pills, many actually start at the time of leaving the hospital. This is also true for progestin-only pills, the pill of choice for women who are going to breast-feed their babies. Pills may be given immediately after an elective abortion performed in either the first or second trimester. OCs may also be started immediately after a premature delivery.

After a woman has completed a full-term pregnancy and started on the oral contraceptives, she must have a follow-up appointment. Traditionally, this appointment was scheduled six weeks postpartum. However, a number of studies have shown that almost half of nonlactating women will ovulate before this time. Therefore, it is increasingly recommended that the postpartum visit be made at three weeks if contraception is not started at the time of delivery. Follow-up visits for young, healthy nonlactating women may be scheduled for every twelve months; however, many clinicians feel that a visit after one or two months of pill-taking is advisable to be sure that the woman is taking her pills correctly, so that she will have an opportunity to ask questions, and so that her initial counseling will be reinforced. Blood pressure should be taken at each visit, and breast and pelvic exams should be carried out on a yearly basis.

Missed Pills

Studies have shown that many OC users frequently miss pills. This phenomenon is particularly prevalent in adolescent OC users. The current approach most clinicians favor is to tell a woman that if she has missed one pill to take that pill as soon as she realizes that she has missed it, and then take the next pill as she normally would. However, if two pills are missed during the first two weeks, she should be advised to take two pills on each of the next two days; some health-care providers recommend using a backup form of contraception, usually a barrier method such as the male latex condom for the next seven days. If two pills are missed in the third week, a backup method should be started as soon as this is recognized. The backup method should be continued for the next seven days, and a new package of pills should be started immediately. If the woman who started her pills on a Sunday misses two pills, she should take her pills every day until the next Sunday and then start a new package.

There is no evidence that using low-dose pills has increased the likelihood of pregnancy in the event of missed pills when compared with rates found with high-dose OCs. Actually many have debated whether or not these missed-pill recommendations are totally necessary. Even women who have skipped four consecutive pills have not ovulated. In another group of women, the pill-free interval was extended for more than one week and, again, no ovulation occurred. However, until additional studies have been carried out looking at the number of missed pills and at the time in the cycle when they were missed, it is probably prudent to continue with the current guidelines to protect the vast majority of women.

Pill Switching

Sometimes switching from one oral contraceptive to another is indicated because of unacceptable side effects. In the case of the monophasic and multiphasic pills, users may start a package of the new pill in place of the original one, keeping to the same general schedule. A switch from a combination pill to the minipill is best accomplished at the end of the original pill package with no time in between.

Use at Perimenopause

Another new question has now arisen as more women are continuing their OCs up to the time of menopause. How does a woman know when she may switch from her use of oral contraceptives to hormone replacement therapy (HRT)? Several ways have been suggested. First, because the average age of menopause has most recently been calculated to occur at 51.4 years, a woman could reach that time and then empirically move to HRT. Additionally, in the *Guinness Book of World Records*, the oldest spontaneous pregnancy was reported at the age of fifty-seven. For those wishing a more scientific approach, past recommendations have been that a woman should stop use of her OC for variable lengths of time, often for about six weeks, using a nonhormonal contraceptive method during that time, and then have a test performed for follicle stimulating hormone (FSH), a pituitary hormone responsible for ovulation. If the result is at or above the level expected in the premenopausal woman, she can then be switched to HRT. However, this approach is now less often advised because of the wide variations that have been found in FSH levels when they are tested in the same woman at different times.

An advantage of older women continuing the use of the low-dose OCs is the fact that without it, they very often experience problems with irregular and heavy bleeding and also tend to have episodes of amenorrhea (absence of menstrual periods) as they approach their menopause. Use of the pill tends to help to reduce or eliminate these problems.

Noncontraceptive Health Benefits

In the earlier publications on OCs, writers tended to begin with long and often very complicated discussions about the potential adverse effects of the pill, particularly on the cardiovascular system. Only after this lengthy discussion was any mention made of the numerous beneficial effects of the pill beyond its high level of effectiveness. Even then, this section usually dealt primarily with the salutary effects that the pill had on certain aspects of the menstrual cycle. Today, with the greatly increased knowledge about the OCs, such a presentation is no longer appropriate and, in fact, is probably counter-productive. Moreover, many people find it ironic and/or inappropriate that while certain warnings about high-dose pills were—and to some degree still are—in low-dose OC labeling, the noncontraceptive health benefits stemming from the use of the oral contraceptives only began to appear in the patient labeling in 1990, although the evidence of these benefits had been around for years.

Ovarian Cancer

Some of the most valuable information gained in recent years through multiple studies on the oral contraceptives has been the collection of data pointing out the steadily growing number of important noncontraceptive health benefits stemming from their use. Probably the most significant finding is that related to the decrease in the risk of ovarian cancer. This malignancy, although not as common as that of cancer of the endometrium, is particularly lethal. In 1998, 25,400 American women developed ovarian cancer and 14,500 died from the disease. It ranks fifth in cancer deaths in women and has the highest mortality rate of any of the gynecologic malignancies, primarily because very few women experience any warning signs during the early stages of this disease. In more than 70 percent of victims, symptoms appear only when the tumor has spread beyond the ovary; at that point the chance of a five-year survival is only about 40 percent. Frighteningly, there is no reliable way at the present time to make an early diagnosis of this disease before it has spread.

Although this cancer begins to appear in women in their thirties, there is more than a tenfold increase in the incidence between the thirties and the mid-sixties. A number of risk factors have been identified. Among these are a family history of the disease, either having no children or a small number of pregnancies, and age, race, and nationality. Many believe that ovarian cancer is related to what is known as "incessant ovulation," women having constant ovulations occurring throughout the majority of their reproductive years. This is in sharp contrast to the many years spent by their ancestors when ovulation was infrequent since women at that time were usually pregnant, lactating, or dead at an early age. Because OCs block ovulation, they may account for the sharp decline in the frequency of this disease seen in women who take them.

There are four major types of ovarian cancer. All of these have been shown to be reduced in incidence by the administration of the various oral contraceptive products including the low-dose pills. After seven years of OC use, there is between a 60 to 80 percent reduction in risk. Even short-term use of the pill shows some level of protection; however, the longer the pill is taken, the greater is the protection that it confers. Finally, it has been noted in a number of studies that this protective effect lasts for at least fifteen years after a woman stops the pill.

Ovarian Cysts

Oral contraceptives also protect the ovaries from certain benign conditions, particularly the development of functional ovarian cysts, both corpus luteum and follicular cysts; the risk in some studies is reduced by as much as 65 percent. However, this protection lasts only during the time the pill is being taken and is due to the suppression of ovarian activity—follicular development and ovulation.

Endometrial Cancer

A second gynecologic malignancy, the most common in women, is endometrial cancer. Recent year 2000 cancer estimates suggest that there will be 36,100 new cases and 6,500 deaths. Endometrial cancer occurs in three major forms, adenocarcinoma, adenoacanthoma, and adeno-squamous carcinoma. Women using the oral contraceptives for a year or more have shown a decreased risk of all three types of endometrial cancer, with the overall risk reduction around 50 percent. As in the case of ovarian cancer, the level of protection has been shown to increase with longer duration of use, being 10 percent at one year, 40 percent at two years, and 60 percent after four or more years. It is currently believed that the progestin in the oral contraceptives is the agent most responsible for lowering the risks of endometrial malignancies and that the protection increases with increasing progestin doses. The protection is greatest in women who are at the highest risk for endometrial cancer—those women who were younger than average when they began to menstruate, those women who have never been pregnant or have had only one or two children, and those who have a late menopause. As in the case of the ovary, protection persists for at least fifteen years after stopping use of the pill. This is particularly important since about 95 percent of these cancers are diagnosed in women in their forties or older.

The prophylactic effects of OCs represent the first time in medical history that a product has been shown to significantly reduce women's risks for two common and frequently fatal malignancies.

Breast Disease

OC users may also protect themselves against other health problems—for example, the development of benign changes in the breasts. Women in all age groups have shown a lowered incidence of fibrocystic disease and fibroadenomas after a year or two of OC use. This protective effect increases with continued use and with increasing doses of the progestin. The protection lasts for at least one year after stopping the pill.

Tubal Disease

Two diseases affecting the fallopian tubes are also less common in OC users. The first of these is salpingitis as part of pelvic inflammatory disease (PID). This condition is a significant contributor to morbidity in women, both acute and chronic disease often leading to subsequent infertility and on occasion, even death. A large study carried out by the Centers for Disease Control and Prevention (CDC) indicated a 50 percent reduction in the risks of hospitalization for PID in OC users; other studies showed a 70 percent reduction in the incidence of PID after one year of OC use. The protection offered by the pill in this case is likely the result of changes in the cervical mucus detailed elsewhere, caused by the progestin in the oral contraceptives.

The second significant major benefit is the almost complete protection against tubal (ectopic) pregnancy, also a significant source of morbidity and mortality in women. Ovulation, particularly with the combined pills, is almost completely stopped, making tubal pregnancy impossible.

Menstrual Problems

Early in the study of the oral contraceptives, researchers recognized that pill use had a salutary effect on a number of the events in a woman's life related to her menstrual cycle. Women with irregular or excessive menstrual bleeding or bleeding between periods often find that the pill regulates both the time frame of their cycles and the amount of bleeding that they experience. OCs have also been shown to be of benefit in the prevention and treatment of excessive blood loss including that seen in women suffering from iron deficiency anemia. This particular benefit may, in some instances, continue even after the oral contraceptives are stopped.

Another condition that affects many women is mid-cycle pain, or *mittelschmerz*. This is believed to be related to the time of ovulation; because ovulation does not occur with pill use, this symptom tends to disappear with OC administration. Pain at the time of menses, dys-menorrhea, is also probably related to ovulatory cycles. Dysmenorrhea is incapacitating for many women, particularly teenagers. Studies of this condition have reported close to sixty percent of teenage girls experience menstrual pain; 10 to 15 percent of that group have missed school because they were incapacitated.

A number of studies have shown that premenstrual syndrome (PMS) is less common and less severe in women using the oral con-traceptives. They report about a 30 percent reduction in the incidence of some of the symptoms of PMS including headache, fatigue, anxi-ety, nervousness, irritability, and depression.

Endometriosis

Use of the pill also helps to protect against such serious medical con-ditions as endometriosis, in which tissue similar to that lining the uterus, the endometrium, is found in the pelvic cavity. This tissue responds to the changes in the hormones of the normal menstrual cycle and mirrors the activity of the endometrium. At the time of the menses, this tissue also bleeds, at which point blood goes into the pelvic and abdominal cavities, producing progressive damage. Endometriosis is currently increasing in frequency and is responsible for considerable pelvic and lower abdominal pain, and pain during sexual intercourse. It is a frequent cause of infertility.

Uterine Fibroids

There are a number of other medical conditions which may also be helped by the use of the oral contraceptives, although the statistical significance of the data relevant to some of them is still somewhat controversial. One of these is uterine fibroids. Protection seems to increase with duration of use. One study reported a 30 percent reduction after ten years of OC use. Fibroids are a frequent cause of hospitalizations and surgical procedures and may, in some instances, contribute to infertility. There is no evidence that the oral contraceptives are useful in the treatment of preexisting fibroids; however, they may confer a protective effect against their future development.

Rheumatoid Arthritis

Some researchers have also suggested that OC use will protect, at least to some degree, against the development of rheumatoid arthritis. Whether this is truly a benefit of OC use or not has been debated for years. One study showed that the risks were decreased by 60 percent and that this effect was most evident in those women who had a strong family history of the disease; other studies have revealed little or no effect. One suggestion has been that the pill may not actually prevent the development of rheumatoid arthritis, but that it may slow the progression of the disease.

Toxic Shock Syndrome

There has been considerable controversy over whether or not there is a correlation between OC use and a decrease in the risk of toxic shock syndrome (TSS). Some studies have reported as much as a 50 percent reduction; others have not shown any beneficial effects. Inasmuch as this disease was originally described in women using tampons of high absorbency, one theory has been that the decreased bleeding seen in OC users may actually be explained by changes in tampon usage.

Osteoporosis Prevention

One of the more recently claimed benefits of OC use is a reduction in bone loss, possibly leading to a decrease in the risk of postmenopausal osteoporosis. This disease and the subsequent development of fractures are common causes of morbidity and mortality in older women. So if the recent claims are true, OC use could provide a major bone-health benefit. If this finding continues to be confirmed, it could have a major impact on women and OC use might help to reduce the more than 1 million fractures that they experience each year.

For a time, the evidence of protection against osteoporosis was controversial. Some studies suggested that the protection against bone loss persisted for only one or two years after discontinuing use of the pill. However, in recent years, a number of additional studies have shown a significant degree and possibly a longer duration of protection against low bone mineral density. For example, one study showed that those women in their fifties and sixties who had used OCs for six or more years had greater bone density in their spines and femurs than nonusers.

Colorectal Cancer

A recently described health benefit is the still debated question of whether OC offers protection against cancer of the colon and the rectum. The Nurses Health Study found that there was a significant degree of protection, which increased with duration of use; however, many of the women in this study had taken high-dose pills. It remains to be seen in future studies whether this protection is also obtained with low-dose pills.

Alzheimer's Disease

It appears that OC use may lead to a reduction in the incidence of Alzheimer's disease. Current research is documenting interesting and perhaps very important evidence of the effects of estrogen on brain tissue. Given the steadily increasing frequency and the lack of effective treatment for this devastating disease, confirmation of these early findings could be a matter of immense significance.

Hormonal Effects of Oral Contraceptives

Reproductive Tract

Because the tissues in the female reproductive tract are the primary targets of the hormones in OCs, changes in these tissues are to be expected.

Vagina   Whereas progestins decrease the amount of vaginal secretions, estrogens produce an increase. Some women are particularly sensitive to estrogens and develop a considerable amount of discharge. This was particularly true when the sequential pill which had several days of unopposed estrogen was being used. Many women have incorrectly interpreted this increase in their secretions as a vaginal infection.

Cervix   For many years the medical community has known that use of the oral contraceptives produces significant changes in the cervix. It often becomes slightly enlarged due to an increase in its blood supply and to overgrowth of its glandular tissue. This produces a clinical condition known as polypoid hyperplasia. There are also predictable changes in the cervical mucus under the influence of the progestin. The mucus becomes very thick and tenacious, blocking the migration of both sperm and bacteria upward through the endocervical canal into the uterine cavity.

There continue to be major controversies regarding the possible induction of malignant changes in the cervix by the use of the oral contraceptives. Attempts to address this issue have shown that there are many different factors involved, which makes finding an accurate answer to this question very difficult, particularly as regards the well-known association of cervical abnormalities with sexual behavior. Factors that increase the likelihood of a woman's developing cancer of the cervix include smoking, the age at which she begins to have sexual intercourse, the number of partners that she (and her partner[s]) has had, and whether or not condoms or female barrier contraceptives—which are known to be protective against cervical cancer—are used. The most important factor, and the one now recognized as the major probable cause of this malignancy is a sexually transmitted disease, human papillomavirus (HPV). The evidence that HPV is primarily responsible for cervical cancer is steadily mounting. HPV is the most common STD in the United States, with an estimated 5.5 million cases diagnosed each year. This infection has now been shown to be caused by more than one hundred different viruses, each of which has now been assigned a specific identification number. Four types are closely linked to cervical cancers. These are types 16, 18, 30, and 45—of these, 60 percent of the cancers are linked to type 16.

This infection is particularly problematic because it is very often asymptomatic. Unfortunately, OC use will not protect against the transmission of this disease. Moreover, there is new evidence that chlamydial infections may also be causative.

There have been a number of interesting but somewhat confusing observations made in efforts to prove whether or not a link exists between pill use and cervical cancer. Women who select the oral contraceptives have been found to have a higher incidence of cervical dysplasia (a premalignant condition) than women who elect to use barrier contraceptives and IUDs. An area of possible influence on this question is the fact that women using OCs generally have better medical care including the frequent taking of Papanicolaou smears, which would allow the early detection and treatment of premalignant changes.

When smoking and other predisposing factors are involved, the evidence for an actual increase in this malignancy due solely to the pill is unclear. For example, several studies of the possible impact of cigarette smoking on cervical cancer have shown that the risk is two to three times greater in smokers as compared to nonsmokers. Furthermore, OC users have been found to have higher rates of smoking than nonusers.

At present, there is no definitive answer to the question regarding the possible adverse effects of the OCs on the cervix. Of perhaps greatest importance is the fact that long-term studies looking at the prior use of the OCs have shown no increase in cervical cancer, which would be expected if a true cause-and-effect relationship existed.

Uterus　There have been many studies on the effects of OCs on the uterus, particularly the endometrium. Estrogens have been shown to increase the amount of endometrial tissue. Progestins, on the other hand, induce progressive thinning of the endometrium and cause it, within about three pill cycles, to go into a resting phase. Cessation of oral contraceptive use leads to the return of the normal pattern of the endometrium, usually within one to two months.

In general, as noted elsewhere, the amount of bleeding seen in women taking OCs is decreased, sometimes progressing to amenorrhea. It is sometimes suggested that this may in fact decrease the risk of infections with certain STDs since these organisms are less likely to proliferate if the bleeding is decreased in amount and duration, as blood is a well-recognized bacterial nutrient.

Fallopian Tubes   It has been hypothesized that oral contraceptives may change the tissues of the tubes and their motility. However, whether this is true or not remains unclear. What is well documented, as already mentioned, is the decrease in morbidity and mortality related to two types of tubal disease. The first is the lowered frequency and decreased severity of certain types of pelvic inflammatory disease, and the second is the virtual absence of ectopic pregnancy due to the suppression of ovulation.

Ovaries   With the continued administration of the oral contraceptives, the ovaries gradually decrease in size. The growth of follicles leading to ovulation is stopped. At one time, it was feared that blocking ovulation over a considerable period of time might result in fertility long after the time when it would normally have ceased. However, the documentation of the fact that follicular development continues during OC use has put this particular concern to rest. In studies carried out to look at the number of eggs found in the ovaries of OC users and a comparable group of nonusers, the numbers were found to be roughly the same. Thus, there is no longer any fear of women having large numbers of "menopause babies." At one time, it was believed that multiphasic pills might have less of an effect in suppressing follicular development than monophasic preparations. However, continued studies have not shown a consistent pattern in this regard.

As previously noted, the use of OCs markedly reduces the risk of ovarian cancer, both during use of the pill and for a long period of time thereafter. However, questions regarding the possible stimulation of benign ovarian cysts persist. In general, there is a decreased frequency of functional cysts; the high-dose pills have a slightly greater effect than the low-dose pills. The possible association of follicular cysts and oral contraceptive use, as measured by hormone assays and vaginal ultrasound examinations, has shown that the single most important factor is the total amount of hormone present in the particular OC a woman is taking.

Breasts

The functional part of the breast consists of a large number of milk glands surrounded by muscular tissue that can contract to express milk through six to eight milk ducts. These structures are encased in a variable amount of fatty tissue. With one small exception, breast tissue is not active until puberty, at which time it starts to develop under the stimulation of estrogen. The exception is the temporary leaking of milky fluid from the breasts of newborn female babies, which is sometimes referred to as "witches' milk" and is caused by the high levels of estrogen the mother produces during her pregnancy.

As part of sexual maturation, a young girl's breasts increase in size and also pigmentation of the areola (nipple area) begins. When progesterone is produced in the second half of the normal menstrual cycle, there is an increase in the activity of the glands. The amount of fluid secretion goes up, and this is what is responsible for the premenstrual breast tenderness that a number of women note. Similarly in oral contraceptive users, under the stimulus of the hormones, some women experience tenderness, pain, and swelling of the breasts. However, these symptoms tend to be most common in the first few months of use, and thereafter they are much less of a problem. Also lowering of the hormonal dose in the OCs has decreased the incidence of significant discomfort. Treatments recommended for those women for whom this continues to be a major problem include a reduction of caffeine consumption and, if necessary, the use of mild diuretics.

Galactorrhea (persistent flow of breast milk) has been noted on occasion in women taking oral contraceptives; this symptom also usually diminishes with increasing duration of use but may continue for a variable period of time after discontinuation of the pill. It is important that this particular symptom be carefully evaluated since it may be the presenting sign of a breast tumor, a tumor of the pituitary gland, or thyroid disease.

Gastrointestinal (GI) Tract

Some women, particularly early in the use of the oral contraceptives, develop nausea with occasional vomiting. These symptoms are possibly due to the action of the estrogen on the center in the brain responsible for vomiting. With continued use, these problems tend to disappear, but if they don't, they are often alleviated by taking the OCs along with food and particularly by timing pill taking to just before bedtime. One practical consideration, if this becomes a significant problem, is that when vomiting occurs shortly after the ingestion of the pill, an adequate amount of hormone may not be retained to block ovulation.

Some experiments have shown that when significant upper GI problems exist, it is possible to administer the oral contraceptives by placing the pills high up in the vagina. The studies have shown that the hormones are then absorbed into the circulatory system and demonstrate normal contraceptive activity.

Biliary Tract

Liver   As noted elsewhere, studies have shown that estrogens act on the liver to change the metabolism of a number of proteins, some of which relate to blood coagulation. Estrogens also affect the way the liver metabolizes lipids and carbohydrates. OC use is contraindicated for women with significant liver abnormalities. However, if a woman has completely recovered from a prior liver infection, for example hepatitis or mononucleosis, and has regained normal liver function, there is no reason to withhold oral contraceptive usage.

Gallbladder   Oral contraceptives increase the amount of certain lipids in the bile due to the estrogen component. This may account for the fact that there is an increase in the number of gallstones in OC users; a similar increase is found in women during or shortly after pregnancy.

Whereas this complication was once thought to occur only after long-term use of the pill, it has more recently been found to occur usually within the first year of use, with no long-term increase in incidence. It is currently believed that the risk is either minimal or nonexistent and that it is confined to those OC users who are susceptible to gallbladder disease in the first place. The pills used today contain a much smaller amount of estrogen than they once did, a factor that would decrease the probability of a woman's developing gallbladder disease due to OC use.

Endocrine Glands

There have been many tests of endocrine function in women using the oral contraceptives. In general, although certain minimal changes have often been noted, they have not in most instances proved to be of any clinical significance.

Pituitary   The efficacy of the combined oral contraceptives depends on the blockage of the release of the hormonal factors that stimulate ovulation. The newer low-dose pills have been found to be as effective as the older high-dose pills in blocking ovulation. Once use of the oral contraceptives is discontinued, the pituitary returns to its normal functions within a matter of days. However, as noted elsewhere, the return of ovulation is apt to be slightly slower.

Adrenal   Minimal changes have been noted in certain adrenal hormones of women using OCs; however, these changes appear to have no clinical importance and are actually less than those seen during pregnancy. Also, it has been found that OCs decrease the amount of androgens produced by the adrenals; however, these changes do not result in any clinically significant alterations.

Thyroid   Over the years there have been many tests involving possible changes to the thyroid due to OC use. Many such changes have been noted and for the most part they are felt to be due primarily to the estrogen in the pill. However, there are no significant changes in such measurements as basal metabolic rate (BMR) and I-131 uptake (a major test of thyroid function), and overall thyroid function typically remains within the normal range. One or two months after stopping the use of the oral contraceptives, the test results returned to their pretreatment levels.

Central Nervous System

Depression   There have been many studies attempting to evaluate whether or not changes in certain emotional states might be pill-induced. One of the clinical conditions that has received the most attention is depression. Studies have reported the frequency of this symptom variously as increased, decreased, and unchanged.

It was initially unclear as to whether depression fell into the psychological or biologic sphere, or both. Social scientists analyzing depression in oral contraceptive users found that certain women had deep concerns and conflicts about having sex for recreation instead of procreation. These individuals developed severe guilt feelings and became very depressed every time they had to take their pills. A few of them actually switched to an IUD or requested sterilization because these options occasioned only a single episode of guilt. On the other hand, some women reported less depression, particularly premenstrually, when using OCs.

In some instances there appeared to be a possible biologic basis for the depression, most notably decreased levels of pyridoxine, Vitamin B_6. Some women taking the pill reported feeling not only depressed but also lacking in energy, often having concurrent episodes of restlessness and insomnia. It has been suggested that the progestin component of the pill might be responsible for some of these symptoms, since use of the progestins has been shown to make some women feel tired and lethargic. However, other possible causes were identified such as recurrent bouts of hypoglycemia and a nutritionally poor diet, which could also lead to a vitamin B_6 deficiency.

In an attempt to resolve these issues, a placebo study was carried out a number of years ago which showed no greater rates of depression in women taking OCs than in the controls using barrier contraceptives. The only exceptions were those women who had a prior history of severe depression or psychiatric disorders and women who had experienced significant episodes of depression with their menstrual periods or following childbirth. However, mild cases of depression have also been reported in individuals who previously did not have this problem, and the issue still remains somewhat clouded.

Depression in OC users has been treated by the administration of vitamin B_6 and tricyclic antidepressants, without conspicuous or consistent success. Lowering of the progestin dose has been reported to be of value in some instances. On occasion, the oral contraceptive must be stopped either temporarily (as a trial) or permanently, if the depression persists or becomes more severe. At the present time, there is little or no evidence that today's low-dose pills are a major cause of depression in previously emotionally stable women.

Libido One of the most interesting and difficult areas in the evaluation of the pill is the subject of libido. Some women have reported mood changes and changes in their sexual responsiveness with use of the OCs. However, observations of this nature are very difficult to evaluate because they are hard to measure and also because the placebo effect is extremely common.

The complexities involved in evaluating this highly subjective type of reaction are considerable and the results have been quite varied. The majority of studies have reported very little overall change in libido. However, there were some studies that showed a considerable increase in sexual desire and in the frequency of sexual intercourse; whether this was due to the hormones in the OCs or to the removal of the fear of unwanted pregnancy was unclear. About an equal number of studies indicated a sharp decrease in libido; very often, however, this occurred in those women who had expressed sharply conflicted feelings about the use of oral contraceptives prior to starting them.

The difficulties encountered in these evaluations were made very clear in the variable results reported in several articles published in the medical literature. In one classic study it was found that there was a dramatic change in libido each time the color of a particular medication being administered was changed. Another study found that libido was most often decreased in the first year of use, particularly in postpartum women. The authors concluded that the decrease was probably more related to childbirth than to the pill. Finally, a striking example of the difficulties of side-effect evaluation came from a placebo study in which 29 percent of the subjects reported lowered libido, 16 percent developed headaches, and 6 percent complained of increased nervousness.

Skin

Acne The use of the oral contraceptives has also been found to play a role in certain skin conditions.

Acne is a common problem for women, particularly those in the teenage group where almost 80 percent suffer, to at least some degree, from the condition. Acne occurs most often around the ages of ten to thirteen, but in some instances it may continue for five to ten years.

Moreover, even women older than thirty-five years of age do on occasion have severe problems with acne.

The lesions of acne occur as pimples, blackheads, and whiteheads. They are found on the upper part of the body including the chest and neck and, most commonly, the face. Acne is caused when the oil called sebum, which is made at the base of each of the skin pores, becomes clogged. If too much is produced, a plug is formed made up of dead skin and sebum. After blockage has occurred, redness and swelling result. Excessive washing of the skin will not only *not* help acne but can actually make it worse. Squeezing of the lesions also is no help; it can make them worse and often results in permanent scarring.

Moderately successful treatment of acne has often included the use of either local or systemic antibiotics. Retin-A products, and a highly effective prescription medication—Accutane (isotretinoin)—are used for severe acne. However, Accutane has been linked to a number of dangerous side effects in pregnant women, including spontaneous abortion, premature delivery, and many severe birth defects. Therefore women taking this medication are always advised not to become pregnant and are urged to use a highly effective contraceptive—very often the OCs—for one month before and one month after Accutane therapy.

A few women develop acne when starting to use OCs where it has not previously been a problem; however, in most instances, women with a preexisting acne condition find that their skin is considerably better when they begin OC treatment. Estrogens, in general, cause an improvement in acne. On the other hand, progestins have been associated with an increase in acne skin lesions. When women with acne have been studied, it has been determined that almost all of them have some change in their circulating androgens, derived from either their adrenals or their ovaries. Androgen levels tend to fall with use of the OCs because of diminished ovarian function. Since estrogens decrease androgens and their activity, this has been one explanation given for the clinical improvement often seen with use of OCs.

There has been a great deal of debate about the so-called androgenicity of certain of the progestins. While small increases in androgen levels sometimes occurred, none of the masculinizing changes associated with excess androgens were ever observed. Current evidence suggests that the low doses of progestins found in today's most frequently used preparations are insufficient to cause acne.

For many years, drug companies tried in vain to win FDA approval to include in oral contraceptive labeling the fact that OCs often decrease problems with acne. The lack of an approved claim, however, did not discourage the prescribing of the pill for this indication, not only by obstetricians and gynecologists but also by dermatologists who had long recognized the value of the OCs in the treatment of acne. Finally, the FDA allowed this claim for one OC; presumably the same claim will soon be generally applied to all of the others.

Malignant Melanoma   For a time, some researchers believed that the use of OCs increased the risk of malignant melanoma, a lethal skin tumor that is currently one of the most common cancers found in younger American women. This theory came from a study of 18,000 women living in California; fourteen women developed the disease and five cases occurred in the control group. Because the number of cases in the treatment group was statistically significant, this particular report was given considerable medical and media attention. Unfortunately, the study failed to look into the amount of exposure these women had had to the sun—a known risk factor—as a possible contributing cause. Subsequent studies from the United States, Australia, England, and Canada have found no association between this malignancy and OC use, when the impact of sunlight was taken into account.

Chloasma   Another skin condition that can occur in OC users is a known as chloasma or "the mask of pregnancy"—a butterfly-shaped increase in pigmentation of the face. It is related to estrogen, ultraviolet light, or both. In fact, those women who developed this condition during pregnancy are more apt to have it occur during OC use. Up to 5 percent of women developed chloasma when taking the higher-dose pills. However, with lowered estrogen dose, this condition is rarely a problem, and when it occurs, it is usually within a particularly susceptible group—women with darker complexions. Unfortunately, some women who develop chloasma, either in pregnancy or with OC use, do not totally lose the skin discoloration after the pregnancy or after stopping the pill.

Varicose Veins   At one time OCs were also blamed for the production of mild superficial varicose veins, but with continued studies, such claims appear questionable. In fact, some women actually seem to experience a slight decrease in varicosities, but again this has not been proved conclusively.

Superficial varicose veins, particularly of the legs, are extremely common in women. They are not associated with any health risks, and must be sharply contrasted with varicosities of the veins deep in the legs which are clearly associated with thrombophlebitis which, on occasion, may result in a pulmonary embolus, which can be fatal.

Hair Loss   A number of years ago OCs were often blamed for hair loss. This finding has not been documented and thus it is no longer considered to be a matter for concern.

Musculoskeletal System

Studies have also been carried out looking at the possible impact of the use of OCs on muscular function, particularly in athletes. So far no significant changes have been found. Of great recent interest is the possible protection given by the use of OCs against bone loss. As noted under noncontraceptive health benefits, several studies now suggest that OCs may help to protect against bone loss and the development of osteoporosis.

Urinary Tract

Several studies have looked into possible changes in the urinary tract resulting from OC use. A British report published in 1974 suggested that there was an association between OC use and urinary tract infections, in 20 percent of the women studied. It further stated that the frequency of the infections was related to the amount of estrogen in the pill being taken. Other research concluded that the ureters (the tubes that connect the kidneys to the bladder) were dilated by OC use; this effect was cited as a product of the progestin component.

More-recent and better-controlled studies have not supported any such associations.

Hematology

Multiple evaluations of many blood factors have been carried out in OC users, particularly because of concerns related to possible thromboembolic complications. Blood coagulation is controlled by a number of factors that are opposite in function, some favoring clotting and others opposing it. Attempts have been made to look at the possible clinical impact of OC use on clotting problems; however to date, no clear pattern has been established.

Diet

Many assays of vitamins have been conducted in OC users. Although slight alterations in individual vitamins have been documented, none of these appear to have any clinical significance and it is not recommended that women on the pill take additional vitamins as supplements if their diet is already adequate. Finally, evaluations of minerals such as zinc, iron, copper, and magnesium have also been carried out. Again, no clinical importance in the variations seen in their blood levels has been found.

Eyes

Early in the use of OCs, a study reported certain adverse changes in the blood vessels of OC users' eyes. However, it was soon recognized that the publication emanated from a referral ophthalmologic practice, and therefore may very well have been skewed by a significant bias in the patients being evaluated. Subsequently collected data showed that the incidence and types of eye abnormalities were the same before women started their use of oral contraceptives as they were during the time of pill administration.

Women taking OCs usually do not experience any changes in their vision; symptoms of visual loss and blurring are not associated directly with pill use. Should these complaints occur, they must be carefully evaluated because they may be caused by vascular spasm or may possibly indicate an impending stroke.

However, there have been reports that some women may experience swelling of the cornea, which produces a change in the curvature of its surface. Depending on the degree of the change, women using contact lenses may experience visual problems and need to have their lenses reevaluated.

Ear, Nose, and Throat

An interesting observation (but one of limited clinical importance) has been the fact that estrogens decrease the amount of earwax. It has also been noted that nasal mucous membranes swell during pregnancy and with the use of estrogens. However, studies have not found any such changes with the use of oral contraceptives.

Immune System

Studies looking at the impact of OCs on the immune system have been both limited and contradictory, especially with regard to traditional antibody evaluations carried out on women who have rheumatoid arthritis or systemic lupus erythematosus (SLE). Regarding the latter condition, one study noted that a worsening of symptoms occurred only in women given the combined oral contraceptives and therefore, for these women, it has been suggested that the progestin-only pill be taken.

Evaluation of viral diseases such as chicken pox suggested an increase in incidence with OC use, but the clinical implications of this finding are unknown. Even where studies have found increased antibodies to various autoimmune conditions, in all cases OC use has appeared to be unrelated to the various clinical signs and symptoms of women suffering from these diseases.

Reproductive Tract Infections

Many studies have looked into the possible effects of OC use on infections of the reproductive tract, both those that are sexually transmitted and others that are not. However, this research has very often shown remarkably conflicting results, some showing an association, some showing protection, and some showing no connection at all.

These evaluations are extremely difficult to do in a way that will allow their results to be reliable as the basis for advice to women. There are several reasons for the problems in getting valid data. The large number of variables that need to be evaluated include, for example, the number of sexual partners of the study subjects and their partner(s)' partner(s), the frequency and type of sexual intercourse, and whether or not condoms were used along with the oral contraceptives. There is some difficulty in establishing the exact time relationship between the onset of the infection and OC use. Above all, it is impossible to carry out comparative trials in which women are randomly assigned to different methods of birth control or no birth control at all for obvious ethical reasons.

Today the disease of most concern is HIV/AIDS. Several studies have indicated an association, but the majority have not found this to be the case. For example, a study in Kenyan sex workers suggested that there was a higher rate of development of HIV in OC users. However, another evaluation of the same study data found that the confounding variables of poverty, condom use, number of partners, and husbands with multiple partners were key to interpreting the significance of these results, and that after a careful reanalysis of all of these factors only a small increased risk remained.

Additional work has suggested that oral contraceptive use alone will not increase the risk of the transmission of HIV infections; however, it has been found that long-term OC users who had genital ulcer disease were twenty-five times more likely to become infected with HIV than a similar group not using OCs and not having genital ulcer disease. Another major factor in the attempt to make accurate analyses between the use of OCs and HIV infections is the known increased risk of HIV transmission—from two to six times more likely—when other genital infections are present, including bacterial vaginosis and STDs such as herpes. Therefore one frequent assumption has been that if OCs contribute to the development of some of the other pelvic infections, they might indirectly increase the risk of the transmission of HIV. Several studies found that HIV-infected women shed the infectious agents in their cervical and vaginal secretions and that it was possible that this might increase the likelihood of HIV transmission. However, other studies looking at the same clinical situations did not find any such link.

Numerous clinical and laboratory studies have been performed to see if there is a correlation between the use of OCs and certain types of vaginal infections. The conclusions have been contradictory. It appears in some studies that there is a level of protection against trichomonas, but this has not been universally shown to be the case. Data are also conflicting on the possible associations with moniliasis (candidiasis), a very common yeast infection. This disease has been studied in OC users for many years with highly variable results; some studies have suggested an increase, some a decrease, and some no change in prevalence. In general, if this infection occurs in a woman who is taking the oral contraceptives there is no need, based on what we now know, to discontinue their use. However, it has been found in certain very resistant cases that temporary discontinuation of the OCs may help in the treatment of the moniliasis infection.

Another disease that has been studied extensively more recently is chlamydia trachomatis. This is an extremely common infection, and some of the older studies of women using high-dose pills suggested that there was an associated increased risk of contracting this disease. On the other hand, an increase has been found to be either less or completely absent in the more recent studies. It has been well documented that use of OCs produces an overgrowth of the tissue on the surface of the cervix, a condition known as cervical ectopy or polypoid hyperplasia. It has been suggested that the organisms causing chlamydial infections might possibly be able to grow more easily in this type of tissue. Unfortunately, studies have very often been unable to determine which occurred first—OC use or ectopy. It has further been suggested that the presence of this cervical tissue overgrowth may simply make easier to detect the presence of chlamydia. Finally, there is growing evidence that at least one serotype (chlamydia trachomatis serotype G) of this organism may be linked to the development of cervical cancer.

Chlamydial organisms are one of the major causes of pelvic inflammatory disease. Several attempts to evaluate OC use and chlamydial infections of the upper genital tract have found a lowering of the risk, perhaps because of changes the progestins in the OCs induce in the cervical mucus, blocking the ascent of the organisms into the uterus. However, a major problem in the analysis of this particular disease is the fact that it is often asymptomatic or mild and therefore unrecognized. As a result women with this infection are less likely to be identified by hospitalizations for treatment of PID than are women admitted for treatment of PID caused by other more virulent infectious agents.

Menstrual Irregularities

As noted in other sections of this chapter, women using oral contraceptives will very often experience, at least temporarily, a change in their menstrual patterns. This may be one of several types and in some women more than one type of irregularity may occur at different times. The most severe—and the major cause for OC discontinuation—is excessively heavy bleeding at the time of the menstrual period (withdrawal bleeding). Another pattern is mild to heavy bleeding between normal periods, called break-through bleeding. On occasion, there will be less bleeding and temporary or continuous amenorrhea may result during OC use.

Weight

Some women using the oral contraceptives tend to retain fluid, resulting in weight gain. This problem is not common and is usually treated by limiting the amount of salt in the diet, and, when more troublesome, by the use of diuretics. In healthy women, fluid retention represents little risk. However, women who have heart disease or any other medical condition where fluid retention is a threat, must deal with this situation very promptly.

Although weight gain has long been viewed as a possible side effect of OC use, a number of studies have indicated that the majority of women do not have an increase in their weight, and also that as many lose weight as gain weight. Where considerable weight gain has occurred, it is almost universally found to be associated with an increase in food consumption and lack of exercise and not related to use of the oral contraceptives. Also women need to recognize that as they grow older, they tend to put on weight slowly and steadily whether they are using OCs or not.

Lipids

No area of OC research has received more attention than the lipid changes noted over the years with the use of the various preparations. Earlier studies, particularly in the era of high-dose pills, suggested that their use increased the risk of cardiovascular disease, thromboembolic disease, myocardial infarction, and stroke. However, the findings of later research indicated that a previously ignored factor—smoking—was the major cause of these increased risks. Nonetheless, continued evaluations, both clinical and laboratory, of the lipoproteins are ongoing and remain a major area of interest today.

There are a number of lipoproteins but three are usually measured when evaluating the overall changes in cholesterol. The three are high-density lipoprotein (HDL), low-density lipoprotein (LDL), and triglycerides. The two components of the combined oral contraceptives have different effects on lipid metabolism. Generally speaking, estrogens increase HDL, which is believed to be protective. Progestins, on the other hand, tend to decrease HDL and increase LDL, changes that may increase the risk of cardiovascular diseases. However, the overall pattern of changes in lipids varies with the particular preparation being studied and particularly with the potency and dosages of the individual hormones.

Because cardiovascular disease, both with and without the use of oral contraceptives, is now a major area of public health concern, numerous studies have been carried out. These are clinical studies, often conducted on large numbers of women and with the use of many laboratory tests, measuring the various levels of lipoproteins. A number of things have been found to influence changes in lipoprotein levels. Genetic factors are of great importance. Diet, lack of exercise, obesity, and, above all, smoking are other key predictors of whether or not a woman will develop problems in this area. It has been recognized that acute symptoms of cardiovascular disease due to the laying down of plaques in various arteries are quite unusual in women who are in the younger reproductive age group. Therefore, a number of evaluations have concentrated on determining the disease rates in women who have previously used oral contraceptives, particularly those who have used them for prolonged periods of time.

Studies of hormones and cardiovascular changes have also been conducted in female cynomolgus macaque monkeys. This particular primate has metabolic and reproductive patterns similar to those of the human female. The monkeys also develop coronary heart disease when given diets that cause atherosclerosis. Studies showed that even when these animals were given a high-cholesterol diet that would elevate their adverse lipoprotein LDL and lower their protective HDL, they did not have an increase in atherogenic changes in coronary blood vessels when given OCs. In fact, some studies showed a protective effect despite the presumably adverse changes in the blood levels of the animals' lipoproteins.

There have been other significant animal and human studies. Rabbits receiving estrogen had fewer changes in their arteries than a control group. Young women using OCs who had myocardial infarctions were found to have less atherosclerosis than a comparable group of nonusers. There is now good evidence that estrogens act directly on the walls of the blood vessels and certain blood coagulation factors; therefore, evaluations of cholesterol and lipoprotein levels alone will not necessarily be indicative of what may be expected to happen to women using the OCs. Moreover, ongoing studies are suggesting that elevated cholesterol levels are only the beginning and not the end of necessary evaluations. Other factors such as changes in homocysteine, C-reactive protein (CRP), and folic acid levels are increasingly being recognized to be of equal or perhaps even greater importance. Thus, this is clearly a much more complex situation than was originally thought.

The major long-term data show that alterations long considered to be adverse—decreased HDL and elevated LDL—are not associated with increased cardiovascular risk, even after stopping OC use. In fact, changes in these lipids, although almost universally found, are not large; the values, in most instances, fall within the normal laboratory range, and are of limited clinical importance. In addition, the lipid values usually return to baseline levels during the days when no hormone is being taken in the pill cycle. Moreover, the animal studies and some epidemiological data would suggest that there is actually a reduction in the risks of myocardial infarction and stroke in women using low-dose OCs.

For a time, it was suggested that all women undergo routine laboratory testing for lipid levels prior to starting OCs. However, in women with normal family histories and no additional risk factors, this practice was gradually discontinued; it was extremely expensive and in general, did not contribute to clinical management. However, if a woman has a known genetic predisposition to cardiovascular disease, she should be screened and monitored carefully. It is now believed that if a woman with elevated cholesterol can lower her levels to normal through the use of a low-fat diet, exercise, or an appropriate form of medical therapy such as a statin drug (Pravachol or Mevacor), there is no reason for her not to use OCs.

Carbohydrates

There has also been concern that use of OCs might induce adverse effects because of their impact on carbohydrate metabolism. In the era of the high-dose OCs, many tests of carbohydrate metabolism were carried out. In general, it was found that there was an impairment of the glucose tolerance test. In addition, insulin and blood sugar levels were elevated. It was believed that the progestin component of the oral contraceptive was responsible for most of the carbohydrate changes and acted by raising the insulin resistance. However, with the development of the newer low-dose preparations and a repetition of the same types of tests, very few to no changes were found in the various measurements of carbohydrate metabolism. The current assumption is that any minor alterations will have little or no clinical importance.

There are a number of clinical areas that have been investigated in this regard. Short-term studies have shown no deleterious effects of the use of OCs on carbohydrate metabolism. In addition, numerous long-term studies have shown no change in the incidence of diabetes. This was true even in that group of women who had known risk factors for diabetes, and even in the era of the high-dose pills and when the pills were taken for a long period of time.

One group that has received particular attention is women who have had gestational diabetes. These are women who, with the stress of pregnancy, develop abnormal carbohydrate metabolism. This tends to revert to normal soon after delivery. For a time, the prevailing theory was that these women were particularly high risk and therefore should not be prescribed OCs. However, this position has changed. No increase in the incidence of the development of frank diabetes in this group has been found, and therefore gestational diabetes is no longer considered to be a contraindication to the administration of OCs.

Another area of concern has been whether or not to give oral contraceptives to women who have insulin-dependent diabetes. Several studies have suggested that the disease does not progress more rapidly if women use OCs. Also, when looking for certain changes often found in the kidneys and the eyes of diabetic women, no adverse effects were found with the use of the oral contraceptives. Moreover, clinical evaluations of cardiovascular and cerebrovascular disease in this group showed no increase. Therefore, the presence of overt diabetes is not a contraindication to the administration of low-dose OCs inasmuch as there is no clinical or laboratory evidence of potential damage.

Of greater clinical significance are recent studies of pregnancies in diabetic women. It is clear that, to avoid known complications for themselves and their babies, women in this group must plan their pregnancies very carefully and make sure that their diabetes is under maximum control before undertaking pregnancy. Therefore, the use of highly effective contraception such as an OC offers a major advantage, helping women to delay pregnancy until they are in the best condition possible to support it.

Evaluation of Side Effects

A major problem in the evaluation of the apparent side effects of any drug is the extreme variability in the design of the clinical and laboratory studies. For example, it has repeatedly been shown that the manner in which information on side effects is gathered is a key determinate of the outcome of any particular study; the differences in the subjects' responses play a major role in establishing the actual incidence of the side effects.

Reviews of the reports in the medical literature point out that side effect data are usually gathered in one of three ways: symptoms are volunteered by the patients, symptoms are ascertained by general questioning, or symptoms are reported in response to questions aimed directly at eliciting information on particular signs and symptoms. The literature makes it clear that questions asked about specific side effects always generate higher frequencies of these side effects than do questions that simply ask the patients how they felt while using the medication.

Evaluating the possible side effects of any drug therapy necessitates the use of a dual perspective, which is of course a very complex process. From the health-care provider's point of view, a particular treatment is selected because of its presumed usefulness in a certain clinical situation and is therefore given to a patient with specific therapeutic objectives in mind. On the other hand, there are always two types of responses from any patient. The first is the patient's physiological (objective) response to the drug; the second is her psychological (subjective) response related to the taking of any prescribed medication.

The patient's response is, to some degree, predicated upon her expectation of what the drug will do for her therapeutically. However, there are other reactions that are often related to her basic personality, her level of knowledge, and her socio-cultural background. Typically, there will be some general or specific emotional overlay generated by the taking of any medication; this is a factor that must also be assessed when evaluating the total impact of a drug.

Sometimes it is easy to separate the biological from the psychological effects of taking a pharmaceutical agent, but at other times the separation of the two may be extremely difficult, if not impossible. This is particularly true when the drug being prescribed has a potentially strong psychological impact. This is clearly the case with the use of OCs, as they are being taken in order to interfere with one of nature's most basic functions, procreation. For some women this interference can precipitate a highly charged emotional situation. For example, it has been well documented that taking the pill can be traumatic for individuals who come from backgrounds where birth control is considered socially, morally, or ethically unacceptable or those who have husbands or sexual partners who are opposed to contraception. These women may experience considerable stress even though, on an intellectual level, they know that taking OCs is a reasonable and appropriate thing for them to do. This increased stress, in turn, may contribute to the side effects that they experience.

Assessment of Pill Side Effects

The pill was originally perceived to be close to the "ideal" drug—totally safe, totally effective, devoid of significant side effects, readily reversible, easy to use, inexpensive, and temporally unrelated to sexual intercourse. In addition, while taking the pill many women experienced the same sense of well-being that they had during their pregnancies.

As time went on, however, particularly since the pill was being given to millions of healthy young women, it became the most studied therapeutic agent in medical history. Numerous clinical and laboratory evaluations were undertaken in centers all over the world. As a result of these studies, it gradually became clear that the OCs did, in fact, have certain adverse side effects in some women.

Reports of these side effects produced fears, both real and unreal, which were fanned by the extensive national and international media coverage given to the OCs, particularly at the time of episodes such as the well-known deliberately biased Gaylord Nelson congressional pill hearings in 1970. These media-driven events resulted in numerous publications in the lay press, many of which were unscientific, inaccurate, and inflammatory. As would be expected, all of this information and misinformation began to produce considerable anxiety among physicians and their patients. Fewer women started taking the pill and more women discontinued use, resulting in well-documented increases in unwanted pregnancies. These, in turn, led to a rise in elective abortions, either illegally at that time in the United States or legally in other countries where safe abortions could be obtained, given sufficient financial resources.

Once the side effects apparently causally related to the use of the pill were more clearly perceived, multiple studies were undertaken to evaluate them. First of all, certain biological and emotional patterns were identified in untreated women, which were then correlated with the hormonal changes known to occur during the normal ovulatory menstrual cycle. This produced a frame of reference against which to place the signs and symptoms occurring in women taking the oral contraceptives. Among these were pain occurring at the time of ovulation (*mittelschmerz*), premenstrual syndrome (PMS), and certain events associated with menstruation (menorrhagia and dysmenorrhea). When women using the combined OCs, which are known to block ovulation, were studied, it was found that ovulation pain did not occur, nor did many of the symptoms associated with PMS. In addition, their menstrual flow tended to be lighter and their dysmenorrhea often disappeared. Thus, it became clear early in the use of the OCs that these drugs provided a number of ancillary benefits beyond that of being highly effective contraceptives.

A number of studies have looked into the psychodynamics of the use of contraception. While the results of these studies varied in certain details, they found that the most important factor in the development of certain side effects was the basic personality of the individual woman. However, even knowing this, there were many variables in these studies that made the final analysis very difficult.

First, the decision to use fertility regulation measures introduced a self-selection bias; women who were willing to start a contraceptive and were motivated to continue its use were often found to be quite different from noncontraceptors. Second, a number of women had significant conflicts about the use of birth control. While most women felt a new sense of power over their lives and a deep sense of relief because of the removal of their fears about unwanted pregnancies, a few developed acute anxiety about their possible loss of self-identity and femininity, once the possibility of pregnancy was taken away. Finally, it was found that certain women subconsciously rejected the idea of not being fertile.

Reports in the psychoanalytic literature suggested that some women perceived of pregnancy as an atonement for their sexuality; such individuals expected and desired pregnancies as a form of punishment. The use of contraceptives removed this possibility and, in some instances, led to considerable guilt, anxiety, and depression. Other studies found that some women who had a basic aversion to sexual intercourse had been using the threat of pregnancy as a means of avoiding coitus. Once they began to use some form of birth control this excuse was effectively removed. They therefore had to face and deal with the reality that they found sexual activity or their sexual partner(s) unappealing. Still other subjects reported tremendous feelings of personal or religious guilt when they indulged in sexual intercourse at a time when they knew that pregnancy was virtually impossible, feeling that they were consciously blocking their basic obligation to have babies.

The loss of the fear of pregnancy of course led to different reactions in different women. Certain women enjoyed sexual activity during a pregnancy whereas in the nonpregnant state they had a marked aversion to coitus; during pregnancy, since there was no longer any risk, these women could relax and enjoy sex. However, for others, their pleasure in sex was sharply dulled by the removal of the possibility of pregnancy, the fear itself adding excitement to their lovemaking. Interestingly, this same reaction has often been noted in men.

To accurately assess side effects, it is necessary to study a drug not only in large numbers of subjects but also in populations drawn from a wide variety of ethnic backgrounds and lifestyles. In addition, nutritional, social, and educational variables have been shown to have major effects on the outcome of such studies.

Often a new drug is evaluated by comparing its results with those seen in a control or placebo group; for obvious reasons, it is rarely possible to do studies of this type when looking at the oral contraceptives. Also, the placebo effect is well recognized in medicine and can significantly alter study results; as noted in the earlier section on libido, an identical OC given to women with multiple changes in the color of the pill induced a marked alteration in the subjects' libidos. Moreover, it was determined in another study that when women were warned in great detail about potential adverse side effects, they tended to experience them much more often than did women whose counseling was less extensive.

In an attempt to get accurate information on the potential side effects of the pill, many studies have compared women using OCs who have a particular condition with those who do not. These are known as case control studies. While they permit an evaluation of relative risk, it is impossible to use this approach to determine cause-and-effect relationships. Another approach is the use of cohort studies. In this type of evaluation, individuals using a particular medication are monitored over a considerable period of time for any side effects. The least useful approach of all is to look at anecdotal information obtained from single individuals or from very small study groups. In the case of the oral contraceptives, an additional complication in long-term evaluation has occurred because of the fact that many women have not taken the same pill for many years—the dosage has been progressively lowered over time.

In the case of the pill, the subjects of many studies have ranged from healthy, young, nonsmoking women to women in their late thirties and early forties, some of whom have medical problems or smoke heavily. Differences are also observed in those subjects taking other drugs which produce a drug interaction as well as many other environmental factors, all of which have impacted the outcome of pill studies. Finally, even if a side effect does occur in a very small proportion of the population using a drug, this fact will very often not be determined until the product has been FDA-approved and sold and used by very large numbers of individuals.

In summary, despite the fact the pill has been the most studied medication in medical history, the issue of its potential adverse side effects continues to be important and complex.

Possible Adverse Side Effects of Oral Contraceptive Use

Hundreds of evaluations have made the pill the most studied medication ever developed. Originally, it was felt that receptors (target tissues) for naturally occurring estrogen and progesterone were to be found only in the female reproductive tract and the breasts. However, over time, researchers have determined that virtually every tissue in a woman's body has estrogen receptors, and many also have progesterone receptors. Therefore, as one would anticipate, the use of the OCs has profound effects all over the body.

Cardiovascular

Thromboembolism   The earliest areas of concern involved the possible OC causation of cardiovascular disease. In the 1960s, originally in Great Britain and then in the United States, there were reports of thromboembolic disease—blood clots, usually in the legs, breaking off and being carried to the lungs, sometimes resulting in a fatal outcome—in OC users. Long-term studies of OC users have generally reported a two- to threefold increase in the risk of thromboembolic disease. However, the actual risk is difficult to evaluate because such things as a family history of this disease, obesity, and diabetes can complicate the data analysis. In addition, geographic differences have been noted; for example, these conditions are rarely seen in the tropics. Moreover, the frequency of this disease had already begun to go up prior to the advent of the oral contraceptives and it had also been noted to be increasing in men. Many laboratory evaluations have been undertaken looking at changes in the various blood coagulation factors. However, as noted, the relationship of these changes to the actual causation of thromboembolic disease has never been totally clarified.

A small percentage of the general population is known to have a predisposition to thromboembolism because of a genetic abnormality known as the factor V Leiden mutation, which was discovered in 1993. Research has shown that this marker occurs in less than 25 percent of individuals with venous thromboembolic disease. Three other markers—protein C, protein S, and antithrombin III—have been identified, but all are relatively uncommon. It is now believed that the majority of the cases of thromboembolism are unrelated to any known markers. Moreover, it has been estimated that 2 million women on the pill would have to be screened for the Leiden factor in order to prevent a single death from thromboembolic disease and would cost more than $100 million.

Screening for a potential thromboembolic complication at the present time is best carried out by taking a careful medical history and looking for potential risk factors not only in the patient herself, but also in other family members. Part of the counseling of all women starting to use the oral contraceptives is to tell them that symptoms such as pain and swelling of the legs, chest or abdominal pain, headache and unexplained visual disturbances might indicate the development of this complication, and that medical attention should be sought immediately.

There are two clinical situations in which the risk of thromboembolism is known to be increased. The first of these is major abdominal or chest surgery. The increased risk lasts for four weeks postoperatively. During this time OCs should not be taken. If the surgery is elective, the use of the pill should be stopped one month in advance, and another form of contraception should be used. The second situation is prolonged immobilization due to illness or injury. In this case, at least two weeks after the immobilization is over should be allowed to elapse before resuming the use of the pill.

The risk of thromboembolism does not appear to be related to the length of time that the pill has been used and it disappears after stopping the oral contraceptives. Furthermore, it has been shown that the risk of thromboembolic disease is linked to the estrogen dose, being increased when the 50 mcg or higher pills are employed. It is currently believed that there may be a very slight risk of nonfatal thromboembolic disease at doses below 50 mcg; however, this risk is markedly lower than that found with a pregnancy.

Stroke The next major cardiovascular complication to be reported was stroke, both hemorrhagic and thrombotic. Between 85 and 90 percent of strokes are due to blood clotting or thrombosis. The remaining 10 to 15 percent are due to rupture of an artery and are called hemorrhagic strokes. Morbidity and mortality rates are considerably higher with hemorrhagic strokes, which include subarachnoid hemorrhages, the most common type of stroke in young women. The reports on strokes in pill users began to appear in the 1960s and continued into the 1970s. Risks in the various studies were described as ranging from two to four times that in women not using OCs.

When some of the older studies were reviewed, it became clear that two other risk factors for strokes were typically involved—smoking and hypertension. The original data analyses did not take into account the additional risk of cigarette smoking. Reviewing data on OC users reveals that the risk goes up markedly in heavy smokers, particularly those more than thirty-five years of age, elevating the total risk by approximately twenty-two times. Risks were also found to be higher for those women using formulations containing 50 mcg or more of estrogen. More recent, better controlled, and better analyzed studies have shown no increase in the risk of stroke among women who are using the low-dose OCs, including the risk of subarachnoid hemorrhage.

Hypertension is also known to increase the risk of stroke in nonusers as well as users of OCs. This topic is covered in detail in the section on medical considerations. Recent studies have shown there is no correlation between the duration of use of the oral contraceptives and the risk of stroke in hypertensive women, nor is the risk of stroke increased after stopping the use of the pill.

Myocardial Infarction   The third and most recently described cardiovascular complication is myocardial infarction. The earlier reported risk was between two and three times higher for pill takers. More recently, the data from the original studies were reanalyzed and additional studies were carried out. It is now clear that the risk is absent or very small unless additional risk factors are involved such as obesity, hypertension, abnormal lipids, diabetes, and, most important, increasing age and smoking. It is very important to recognize that if one looks at the risks of myocardial infarction, first with increasing age and second with smoking, the combined risk is considerably higher than if the two individual rates are taken separately and then added together, a phenomenon known as synergy. It now appears that there is little or no increase in the risk of heart attacks for women who are using low-dose pills unless they are older and smokers. Finally, recent studies have shown no increased risk of myocardial infarction after women stopped the use of the pill. This last observation is one of great clinical importance.

Hypertension   It is important to check a woman's blood pressure before and during the use of the oral contraceptives. Many women taking OCs have a very slight increase in their blood pressures. However, the pressures obtained are still, in almost all instances, within normal limits. A few individuals will develop significant hypertension, often becoming symptomatic, and this mandates the immediate stopping of the pill, at which point blood pressure will return to normal.

For a time, it was believed that women who had hypertension during pregnancy as part of eclampsia, and women who have a strong family history of high blood pressure should not use the oral contraceptives. However, there is no universal agreement on this point, and neither is currently believed to be an absolute contraindication. The most important factor is continued monitoring of the blood pressure during pill use.

Smoking   As already noted in several other sections, the impact of smoking on the development of cardiovascular complications in both pill users and nonusers is immense. It has long been known that the nicotine in cigarettes increases the heart rate as well as the blood pressure. This results in an increased demand for oxygen on the part of the heart muscle. In addition, heavy and prolonged smoking produces damage to the lungs, which in turn decreases the amount of oxygen getting to the heart. There are numerous clinical signs indicating that someone is highly dependent on the use of nicotine. They include such things as smoking early in the day, heavier smoking in the first part of the day, smoking more than a pack a day, and having had a number of withdrawal symptoms when the person attempted to stop. They also include a craving for cigarettes; an increase in appetite and consequent weight gain; and a number of mood changes including restlessness, anxiety, frustration, anger, depression, insomnia, and difficulty in concentrating.

One of the major contributions that women could make to their health is never to start smoking or, having started, to stop the use of cigarettes. In addition to the well-known complications of lung cancer, cardiovascular disease, facial wrinkling, and many other illnesses and malignancies, it is now clear that cigarette smoking as well as secondhand smoke have a major impact on many body tissues, on reproductive function, and even on unborn children. Two articles, both published in 2000, have added to the reported risks. First, there is an increased risk of breast cancer in women exposed to both active and passive smoking. Second, breast cancer rates are somewhat higher in women who smoked as adolescents. Finally, a new study from the Netherlands has shown a threefold increase in a common skin cancer—squamous cell carcinoma—in smokers. The risk increased as the number of cigarettes smoked went up, going to a fourfold increased risk in those who smoked twenty-one or more cigarettes a day. Individuals cannot be considered to be smoke-free until they have gone at least a year without smoking. Also, women getting nicotine from other sources such as patches and gum, because of their nicotine content, must be considered to be smokers.

Weight gain is one of the key concerns of teenagers. It has been found that many teenagers refuse to take the pill because they believe it will cause them to get fat, and they smoke in order to keep their weight down. Even if they start OCs, they often continue to smoke for the same reason.

Many educational materials, such as flip charts, videotapes, and instructional brochures, have been developed, all aimed at helping people to stop smoking and to remain smoke-free. It is unfortunate and somewhat remarkable, given the amount of information on the adverse effects of smoking, that this question is not routinely asked of all potential pill users. Even when antismoking advice is given, follow-up counseling sessions are not always made available.

Despite the admonition against giving the oral contraceptives to women over the age of thirty-five who smoked, one survey showed that about a quarter of the women in this age group taking the pill were continuing to smoke. In fact, 85 percent of this group smoked more than fifteen cigarettes per day, a fact which classified them as heavy smokers. The data suggest that these women may not always be totally open when they give their medical histories and request the use of the pill.

Women under the age of thirty-five who are heavy smokers may be considered candidates for OC use if this is their method of choice for other good reasons. Although the risk of cardiovascular complications exists, it is relatively low in this age group. Moreover, the decreasing amounts of estrogen in the pill have made the usage more feasible.

Breast Cancer

Now that many of the concerns about OCs and cardiovascular disease have been at least partially put to rest, the biggest area of controversy today is the possible association between the use of the oral contraceptives and breast cancer. Many reports have been published over the years, some of them being extremely contradictory. At the present time, there is no indication that oral contraceptives will initiate the occurrence of breast cancer. However, a theory still exists that they might stimulate the earlier development of this disease in women who already have premalignant tissue.

More than half a million women in the United States have cancer of the breast, and there are 43,300 deaths every year. The American Cancer Society estimated that there would be 175,000 new cases in 1999; the estimate for 2000 was 183,000 cases. By the time a woman reaches the age of sixty, she has a lifetime risk of being diagnosed with breast cancer of approximately 10 percent. This figure is often misinterpreted as meaning that one in ten women will develop breast cancer, but actually it only means that there is a 10 percent chance of being diagnosed in the older age group. This disease is much less common under the age of thirty-five and increases between the ages of thirty-five to forty. Following this, it continues to increase very slowly, with more than 80 percent of the cases found in women over fifty years of age.

A number of factors may be involved in increasing the risk of developing this disease with oral contraceptive use. These include the age of the individual, the age at which she began to have menstrual periods, the age at which she began to use the OCs, the type of pill and the dosage that was used, duration of use, family history of breast cancer, racial background, height, weight, alcohol use, and smoking. Other studies have indicated that certain factors decrease the risk of breast cancer. These include removal of the ovaries prior to menopause, a first pregnancy at an early age, and the onset of the menarche at a later age. In addition, preliminary data suggest that no increase in breast cancer has been seen with OC use since 1975, possibly because of the much lower doses of estrogen and progestin.

There is a general rule that when an association exists between a drug and the induction of a specific disease, increasing duration of use and increasing dosages will tend to be correlated with an increase in the incidence of that disease. This has never been shown to be true in the case of the oral contraceptives and the development of breast cancer, suggesting a lack of causation.

The largest epidemiological study ever conducted on the possible association was done by the Collaborative Group on Hormonal Factors in Breast Cancer. This study collected information on more than 53,000 women with breast cancer and 100,000 controls. Data were gathered from fifty-four studies conducted in twenty-six countries. Two analyses of the data from this study were published in 1996. They led to the conclusion, first, that women currently using the pill and those who had taken the pill within the past ten years had a small increased risk of being diagnosed with breast cancer. Second, there was no significant increase in the risk in women diagnosed ten or more years after discontinuing the use of the oral contraceptives.

The study report suggested that the diagnosis of breast cancer might be more apt to be made in women taking the oral contraceptives because they are receiving more comprehensive medical care. However, when tumors were found, they were more often noted to be limited to the breast tissue, possibly because their cancers were diagnosed earlier than might have been the case otherwise or, alternatively, that use of the OC actually affected the growth of the tumor itself and its tendency to spread. The study also indicated that up to twenty years after stopping the pill and comparing women who had and had not used the oral contraceptives, there was little difference in the total incidence. Moreover, when OCs were started in both younger women and older women there was no difference in the risk of breast cancer. Other studies have shown conflicting data on long-term OC use prior to a first pregnancy; in some studies, a small risk was noted, however, in others no association was found.

Two other very large studies were conducted, the first by the CDC, and the second by the Royal College of General Practitioners. In both cases, there was no increase in the risk of breast cancers in OC users. In the Nurses Health Study, long-term health data on 118,000 female nurses were evaluated. There was no evidence that the past use of OCs was associated with an increased risk. Additional data indicated a protective effect against breast cancer in women who had stopped the use of the pill at least ten years earlier. It also showed that there was no evidence for an increased risk for women up to the age of fifty-five and no evidence for an increased risk for women with a family history and women who have benign breast disease. The only possible increase, although one still much debated, is a slight elevation in long-term users under the age of forty-five.

The number of cases of breast cancer continues to increase. It is clear that studies will have to be continued to obtain definitive answers as to the possible relationship between oral contraceptive use and this malignancy. However, it is already clear that the risk, if indeed it does exist, is very small and is heavily counterbalanced by the well-established health benefits of the use of these agents, particularly the prevention of ovarian and endometrial cancer. Unfortunately, women continue to be alarmed out of all proportion to the actual danger. A study carried out by the National Cancer Institute (NCI) in 1995 revealed that women thought that their risk of dying from breast cancer was actually twenty-five times higher than the actual statistics!

Clinical Management of Side Effects

Excessive Bleeding

Women who experience heavy menstrual bleeding after the first few months of OC use, can sometimes resolve the problem by changing to a product with more estrogen or a higher progestin potency. Two approaches have been tried in attempts to control the bleeding; neither one was successful. One was to double the number of pills taken when bleeding occurred. This approach did not seem to be of much help and it was confusing, so it was discontinued. The second approach was simply to stop the pills and wait for a menstrual period. This, unfortunately, often ended in an unwanted pregnancy, so it too was discontinued.

Breakthrough Bleeding

Bleeding between menstrual periods is most common in the first one or two pill cycles and tends to decrease with continued use. If breakthrough bleeding is minimal and occurs early in the use of OCs, a woman should continue to take her original medication. By and large, this type of bleeding tends to stop after three to four months of use.

One approach to this problem has been to change the type of oral contraceptive being used. Although abnormal bleeding sometimes appears to be improved on a different preparation, very often what has really happened is that additional time has passed and the bleeding would have stopped in any event. There is no particular pill which is significantly better than any of the other OCs in terms of the prevention of breakthrough bleeding.

A second approach that has been used is the administration of extra estrogen for about seven days while the bleeding is occurring. Very often, this will resolve the problem; however, if bleeding continues, a second round of this therapy may be needed. If bleeding continues and becomes excessive, it is essential to find out the cause and then to deal with it appropriately. The bleeding could be related to a cervical or uterine tumor, either benign or malignant. It could be a sign of an ectopic pregnancy or a missed abortion. It could be due to the development of a hemorrhagic disorder or PID.

Women must understand that breakthrough bleeding does not indicate a failure in the effectiveness of the OC.

Amenorrhea

Amenorrhea occurs in pill takers because there is insufficient estrogen present to stimulate the development of the endometrium; there is less growth not only of the glandular tissue but also of the blood vessels.

Amenorrhea is a fairly common side effect, but if a woman has taken her pills correctly, there is little reason to be concerned about an unplanned pregnancy. However, if the lack of bleeding continues, pregnancy must be ruled out. If amenorrhea poses an emotional problem, very often use of a pill with more estrogen will help until the bleeding cycles are stabilized. Occasionally, a woman will have a prolonged episode of amenorrhea after stopping her use of OCs. In most instances, no immediate treatment is necessary since eventually menses do return to normal in almost all cases.

The lack of withdrawal bleeding is disturbing to both the women using the pill and the health-care providers taking care of them. There are two major considerations. First, this may represent an early pregnancy and although, as noted elsewhere, there is no evidence of any damage to a developing fetus from OC use, it remains a concern both emotionally and medicolegally. If pregnancy is a possibility, one of the currently available highly sensitive diagnostic tests for early pregnancy can be used. However, if amenorrhea becomes a recurrent problem, repeating pregnancy tests can be not only expensive but also disconcerting. A much simpler way to establish the presence or absence of a pregnancy is to use the basal body temperature. This should be done by the woman at the end of her pill-free period of time or after she has taken the last of the pills which contain no hormones. If her temperature is less than 98 degrees Fahrenheit, this means that she is not pregnant and she can continue the use of her OCs. However, if her basal body temperature is above 98 degrees Fahrenheit, pregnancy is a possibility and therefore she should have a pregnancy test.

Some women are concerned that the development of amenorrhea means that their endometrium will not regrow, and that their ovaries and uterus will not return to normal and permit future pregnancies. They need to be reassured that no permanent damage will result from an episode of amenorrhea. To relieve their fears, some clinicians add additional estrogen during the hormone phase of the pill cycle. This allows for a buildup of more endometrial tissue and as a rule will produce withdrawal bleeding. This approach is often successful, and no further episodes of amenorrhea may be noted for several months.

Nausea and Vomiting

Some women taking the OCs develop nausea. This complication is most common in the first few months and usually disappears with continued use. There are several ways of dealing with this adverse side effect. Taking the pill with food is often helpful; even more effective is taking the pill at bedtime so that the nausea occurs during sleep and is unnoticed.

Occasionally, nausea will progress to actual vomiting. A concern in this regard is that if excessive vomiting occurs frequently, insufficient amounts of hormone will be absorbed, ovulation may not be blocked, and therefore pregnancy becomes a possibility. Very often the administration of an antiemetic drug helps to relieve these symptoms if they continue and are severe.

Breast Changes

Tenderness of the breasts is very common early in OC use and tends to disappear with continued use. It is due to the estrogen component of the pill. Some women also note enlargement of their breasts, the result of fluid retention caused by the hormones, a change which they may or may not find desirable.

Another problem that has occasionally been noted is galactorrhea—the excessive or persistent flow of milk from the breasts. While in some individuals this may be related to use of OCs, as noted elsewhere, it is often a sign of thyroid disease or the development of a pituitary microadenoma. Therefore, the presence of galactorrhea always mandates a careful medical evaluation.

Headache

Headaches are a very common complaint; in fact, some reports estimate that they are the seventh leading reason for visits to emergency rooms. Close to 100 percent of women report having headaches at some time and up to half at fairly frequent intervals. Therefore it is extremely important to be able to evaluate headaches when considering not only whether or not to start OCs for a particular woman who report having headaches but also whether or not to discontinue their use by women because of the development of headaches during treatment.

It is important to be able to classify headaches correctly. Factors of major diagnostic significance are the type of headache; when, where, and how often they occur; their severity; and whether or not there is a family history of this condition. Headaches fall into four major categories, although more than one type may occur at different times in any individual woman.

Tension Headache   These are by far the most common type of headache. They are usually described as dull and constant although their severity may vary. The pain is usually bilateral and is perceived as a tight bandlike sensation around the head. Very often they are accompanied by tightness and pain in the neck and shoulder muscles. They are most often associated with stress, emotional problems, anxiety, and depression. They tend to recur and to last for a considerable period of time.

On physical examination and with further diagnostic testing, no specific cause can be found for such headaches. They are best treated by reassurance and pain relief with the use of aspirin, acetaminophen, nonsteroidal anti-inflammatory drugs, and muscle relaxants.

Migraine Headache   Migraine headaches are of two major types, first those without an aura (a warning sensation that precedes the development of one or more neurological symptoms), also known as common migraine, and second, those with an aura, also called classic migraine. Twice as many women as men experience these headaches, and there is often a family history.

Common migraine is the more frequently seen. It is usually bilateral, throbbing in character, and is often accompanied by heightened sensitivity to light and sound and by nausea, vomiting, and loss of appetite. These headaches can be triggered by certain foods, alcohol, missing meals, fatigue, and changes in the weather.

Classic migraine headaches are usually unilateral and throbbing in character. They differ from common migraine in that they are accompanied by neurological signs such as loss of visual fields (scotomata) and flashing lights or spots (scintillating scotomata). These symptoms tend to occur just before the attack, increasing over a period of five to twenty minutes and lasting for up to an hour. There may also be dizziness and weakness on one side of the body. All these neurological complaints go away when the headache stops. Women with this type of headache report the same sensitivities, gastrointestinal symptoms, and triggering causes as those experienced by sufferers of common migraine.

Migraine headaches also occur in women using OCs. Some with previously existing migraine find their symptoms are improved, others are made worse, and a few will develop symptoms for the first time when they start to use the pill. It has been shown that women taking OCs who have tension headaches and migraine headaches without any aura are at no greater risk of having a stoke than nonusers. However, women who have neurological symptoms should not be given the pill.

Headache Due to Brain Disease   These headaches are found on examination to be due to some neurological disorder; the causes include brain tumors, strokes, and hypertension. Women with this type of headache characteristically have neurological signs not only during but after the headaches. The pain in these cases is often quite severe and may be accompanied by fainting episodes.

Clinical Management   Headaches that develop while a woman is taking OCs are a major source of concern to both health-care providers and patients. In women who take OCs, headaches may be associated with fluid retention, migraine, or hypertension, but much more often they are related to increased tension in the women's environment. In one interesting and provocative double-blind study, headaches were found to be most common in the cycle immediately prior to the institution of treatment with OCs.

When a woman complains of headaches, it is extremely important to characterize the headache by its location, severity, and duration and to know whether she has had headaches in the past or whether this represents a new symptom since starting treatment with OCs. The type of headache that may be the warning sign of an impending stroke is one that starts with pill use; is accompanied by dizziness, nausea and vomiting, visual symptoms, or hypertension; is severe, of long duration, unilateral; and is unresponsive to analgesics. It is rare to find a woman who has had a stroke who did not have one or more of these premonitory signs, and they are a clear indication for the immediate cessation of OC therapy and for careful evaluation.

Medical Considerations

For a number of years, OCs were viewed primarily as a therapy to be used by healthy young women. However, with the passage of time, it became clear that oral contraceptives might well be used by women who were not completely healthy and by women who were no longer very young. Therefore, much more attention was paid to a number of medical conditions, attempting to determine the risk/benefit ratio of OC use for individuals who had these conditions (see the following section).

The World Health Organization (WHO) in 1996 released suggested guidelines for dealing with these issues, recognizing that agencies, programs, and individual health-care providers often needed additional guidance when dealing with the women who had certain specific diseases. WHO's stated objective was to allow the maximum use of the oral contraceptives without imposing any health risks to women. In order to carry out this objective, a number of international experts from many organizations were charged by WHO with reviewing the relevant medical literature.

Early in the course of this evaluation it became obvious that many of the existing policies and practices were actually based on information drawn heavily from the older literature on high-dose pills. They had found their way into and were still listed inappropriately in the labeling of the low-dose oral contraceptives and did not reflect the information gathered in recent years on various aspects of the use of the newer products. As a result, WHO believed that a number of women who were being denied the use of the oral contraceptives were actually able to take them with a high degree of safety.

Following the completion of this thorough literature review, WHO created a rating scale aimed at giving guidance to OC prescribers. The various medical conditions that had been researched were placed in one of four categories. Category I consisted of conditions where there were no restrictions on OC use. Category II included conditions where the advantages of OC use generally outweighed the risks. Category III listed conditions where the risks of OC use, in most instances, outweighed the advantages; the only exceptions in these cases were the situations in which other more appropriate methods were either not available or were not acceptable. Category IV conditions were those judged to be contraindications to the use of the oral contraceptives.

The following section lists alphabetically a number of medical conditions and reviews their relationship to OC use. Each one reflects the WHO categories plus additional research information that has been gathered since the time of the publication of the WHO report. Many of these conditions are covered in much greater detail elsewhere in this chapter.

Oral Contraceptive Use with Specific Medical Conditions: Risks vs. Benefits

Abortion	Oral contraceptives may be started shortly after either a spontaneous or induced abortion.
Acne	Acne is a condition the prevention of which was, for a long time, not listed as an advantage to OC use. It is now recognized to be an additional indication for the use of oral contraceptives.
Age	It was previously recommended that OC use be stopped at age thirty-five in smokers and at the age of forty in nonsmokers. It is now well recognized that healthy nonsmoking women may use the low-dose OCs safely up to the time of menopause. Smokers over thirty-five, however, still should not receive the OCs because of the high risk of cardio-vascular complications that results from the synergistic combination of OCs and smoking.
Amenorrhea	The absence of menstrual periods may be spontaneous or induced. Women in the spontaneous group need a careful medical evaluation prior to making a decision as to whether or not to use OCs.
	Induced amenorrhea, which occurs as the result of OC use, once pregnancy has been ruled out, is not a reason to discontinue OC therapy in the absence of any other significant abnormality.
Anemia	Anemia may be affected in one of two ways by OC use. First, the prevention or amelioration of iron-deficiency anemia is included among the noncontraceptive health benefits because it has been shown that the use of OCs will, in general, decrease the total amount of blood lost during the monthly flow.

Anemia (continued)	On the other hand, although it is far more rare, excessive bleeding may occur during the administration of the pill causing anemia. This may demand a change in the therapeutic regiment if it continues, and if this does not readily resolve the problem, a medical evaluation is necessary.
Antibiotics/Antimicrobials	Certain medications used in combination with OCs have been shown to interfere with the function of one or both agents, as described in greater detail in the section on drug interactions. Researchers have evaluated a number of antibiotics in recent years in attempts to establish whether or not a drug interaction occurs with the use of the oral contraceptives. In the past some of the tetracyclines and penicillins have been thought to interfere with the efficacy of the OCs. However, the most recent evaluations have not borne this out. These studies have also included the antifungal drug griseofulvin. Women using this agent should use a 50 mcg OC because of a known drug interaction.
Anxiety States	Women suffering from anxiety states may use OCs; in fact, where fear of unwanted pregnancy is a contributing factor, they may be of significant help. However, when tranquilizers such as diazepam (Valium), chlordiazepoxide (Librium), tricyclic antidepressants (imipramine), and theophylline are also being administered, it may be necessary to decrease the dose because of possible drug interactions with OCs, slowing their elimination from the body.
Atherosclerosis	The exact role of OCs in the potential development of this condition remains unclear. There is some evidence that its prevention may possibly be one of the noncontraceptive health benefits arising from the

use of the pill. However, the conclusions about the actual impact of OC use in this area are constantly changing and therefore further studies are still actively being pursued.

Bleeding Disorders

Contraceptive use has been evaluated in a number of bleeding disorders. These include hemorrhagic diseases, coagulopathies, and the various blood dyscrasias. In general, oral contraceptives may be of value in a number of these conditions because they may induce an increase in clotting factors, which would be useful in hemorrhagic states. A specific disorder, von Willebrand's disease, which comprises a group of bleeding disorders, has been found to be helped by the use of OCs. Moreover, at the present time, there is no reason that women who are on anticoagulant therapy should not use the oral contraceptives, unless there is an additional overriding medical problem.

Breast Disease

The significance of a positive family history of breast cancer in determining the risk for a particular woman has been narrowed to women who have first-degree relatives with this disease. Women with active breast cancer should not be given OCs. However, there is a growing body of evidence that women who have been treated for breast cancer in the past and who have gone for five years without any evidence of recurrence may possibly be candidates for OC use.

Prevention of benign breast disease is included among the noncontraceptive health benefits of the use of oral contraceptives. Also women who already have benign breast disease are very often improved after using OCs for several years.

Chloasma	This condition—a darkening of the skin of the face—is a known side effect of oral contraceptive use in certain women. However, it is not felt to be an absolute contraindication.
Depression	Despite early evidence suggesting an association between oral contraceptive use and the development or the worsening of depression, more recent studies on low-dose OC use do not show this effect.
	When antidepressants such as imipramine are being administered, it may be necessary to decrease their doses by one-third if OCs are to be given concurrently. Also Saint-John's-wort, now commonly being used in the treatment of depression, causes the hormones in OCs to be excreted more rapidly and has been thought to lead to breakthrough bleeding.
Diabetes	The subject of OC use and diabetes is covered in greater detail in the section on medical considerations, only a summary being included here.
	Gestational diabetes was at one time considered to be a relative contraindication to oral contraceptive use. However, with the current pills, this condition is not considered to be a contraindication. The WHO guidelines on oral contraceptive use in diabetic women, both noninsulin and insulin-dependent diabetics, suggest that those who do not have any serious cardiovascular complications should be allowed to use the OCs, the risk/benefit ratio in this case most often being on the side of the benefits. However, once cardiovascular disease or other complications such as retinopathy (eye disease) develop, these individuals fall into either WHO Category III or IV. The determining factors as to whether a woman

belongs in Category III or IV depend on two things—
the severity and duration of her particular disease.

Diethylstilbestrol (DES)	DES is a synthetic estrogen that was widely used in the United States and Europe during the 1950s and 1960s in attempts to prevent first trimester spontaneous abortions. In 1971, it was reported to be linked to the development of a certain malignant vaginal tumor in some of the daughters of these women. Considerable research in the intervening years has been carried out to attempt to assess the actual potential dangers of the use of DES and particularly to evaluate whether or not the use of hormones such as the OCs might be contraindicated in these daughters. The most recent review, published in year 2000, suggests that OCs will not increase the risk of a woman developing this tumor if she was exposed to DES in utero.
Dysmenorrhea	As noted elsewhere in this chapter, dysmenorrhea or painful menses is directly related to ovulation. Since OCs block ovulation, considerable improvement in dysmenorrhea is a usual benefit.
Ectopic Pregnancy	There is no reason to deny women who have a history of prior ectopic pregnancy the use of the combined oral contraceptives. In fact, the prevention of ectopic pregnancies is one of the major noncontraceptive health benefits of OC use because ovulation is suppressed.
Endometriosis	This very common disease has been treated with oral contraceptives quite successfully for a number of years. In addition, there is early evidence that the incidence of endometriosis may actually be decreased with the use of these agents, as noted in the section on noncontraceptive health benefits.

Estrogen-Dependent Tumors	The presence of any tumor that has been shown to be stimulated by estrogen is a contraindication to the use of oral contraceptives. In fact, it is labeled as an absolute contraindication to all products containing estrogen.
Family History	While it is always a good idea to get a complete and accurate family history when considering OC use, it is especially advisable under several specific conditions. Probably the most significant family history is that of premature death—death at a young age—of a parent from cardiovascular disease.
Gallbladder	Oral contraceptives may stimulate the production of gallstones in susceptible women. For those who have already had gallbladder disease—for example, a woman with a history of gallstones—oral contraceptives should be given only rarely. Once the gallbladder has been removed, there is probably no reason not to use OCs.
Headaches	Whether or not headaches constitute a contraindication to OC use depends on the type of headache with which a woman presents. The differentiation and management of the various types of headaches are discussed extensively elsewhere in this chapter.
Heart Disease	A woman who is born with congenital heart disease or who develops valvular heart disease must be carefully evaluated when making a decision about whether or not OCs can be used. If this evaluation exposes a condition that might predispose her to a thrombosis of the coronary blood vessels, or if a woman is having severe problems because of a very limited cardiac reserve, these constitute contraindications as does a prior myocardial infarction in most cases.

Women who have a mitral valve prolapse are at increased risk of thromboembolic disease, but only if they are symptomatic. Therefore, particularly in smokers, OC use should be considered in only the most unusual circumstances. However, if the woman's prolapse is asymptomatic, she may use low-dose combined pills or progestin-only OCs.

Hirsutism

The oral contraceptives are often useful in the treatment of hirsutism and thus may be regarded as one of the possible noncontraceptive health benefits.

HIV/AIDS

It is generally believed that there is no reason not to give the oral contraceptives to women who are HIV-infected or who have developed clinical AIDS. Clearly there is a need in most of these individuals for a highly reliable form of birth control to protect against unwanted pregnancy; therefore, oral contraceptives are frequently recommended for this group. However, because OCs do not protect partners from possible infection with the virus, other prophylactic measures, such as the use of condoms, are vital as well.

Hypertension

In general, most clinicians feel that low-dose OCs may be used in women who previously had high blood pressure, provided that they are under the age of thirty-five, are otherwise healthy, and do not smoke.

It is possible that those whose hypertension is controlled by medication can also safely use OCs. There continues to be considerable debate about this, however. Some health-care providers feel that having achieved a normal blood pressure enables these women to use the pill, whereas others believe that the presence of hypertension indicates underlying

Hypertension (continued)	vascular disease and constitutes a relative contraindication.
	The World Health Organization guidelines separate hypertension into three different categories to aid in the decision as to whether or not an individual woman is a candidate for OC use. First, they place women with blood pressures of 140–159/90–99 mmHg in either Category II or III, depending on other risk factors and whether or not careful monitoring can be done. Second, for women with blood pressures of 160–179/100–109 mmHg, WHO recommends starting OCs only if no additional risk factors are present and if a woman is able to have regular careful monitoring of her blood pressure. A blood pressure of 180/110 mmHg places a woman in Category IV and constitutes a contraindication.
	For women using OCs, a blood pressure of 160–179/100–109 mmHg should mandate OC discontinuation. Finally, when antihypertensive agents such as cyclopenthiazide and guanethidine are being used along with OCs, it may become necessary to increase the dose of these agents because of the possible development of a drug interaction.
Infectious Mononucleosis	There is no reason for a woman with this disease not to use the oral contraceptives as long as liver damage has not occurred, and her liver function tests are normal.
Lactation	Women who are either not breast-feeding or are using supplements of formula in addition to breast milk should start OCs at three weeks after delivery. Those who are breast-feeding their babies without additional supplementation should begin at three months.

Lipids

There are a number of genetic hyperlipidemias. If the changes are mild, there is no reason not to use low-dose OCs, as they have no significant clinical impact on blood lipids with the exception of triglycerides, which are predictably increased by the use of estrogen. However, if a woman already has a diagnosis of vascular disease, and particularly if she smokes, OCs may not be the ideal method of contraception. The WHO classification in these cases is either Category II or III depending on the type of hyperlipidemia and also on the severity of the disease. If oral contraceptives are elected, it is important that lipid levels be measured monthly for several months to make sure that there are no clinically significant changes in their levels.

Liver Disease

Women who have cirrhosis of the liver may not be good candidates for OCs. If the case is relatively mild, then OCs may remain an option; however, if there is significant damage, oral contraceptives should not be given.

The presence of active viral hepatitis is a major contraindication to OC use. Women who previously became jaundiced during a pregnancy were at one time believed to be poor candidates for OC use. However, the current view is that this is a less rigid contraindication, provided that the woman is willing to be followed very closely and knows that her pills will be discontinued if it appears that she is developing liver damage.

Lung Disease

Oral contraceptives have no impact on lung disease. However, for a women using a bronchodilator such as aminophylline, it is recommended that the starting dose be reduced by a third if the woman is an OC user. This is due to a known drug interaction.

Mittelschmerz	The pain some women experience at the time of ovulation is usually mild, but in a small percentage of cases may be fairly significant. Because women on OCs do not ovulate, *mittelschmerz* ceases to be a problem for them.
Obesity	A woman who is obese may be given the OCs unless she has other health problems that would contraindicate their use.
Osteoporosis	Osteoporosis prevention is currently being considered as a possible reason to use oral contraceptives, which would add another potential health benefit to OCs' growing list. Moreover, hormonal therapy is often indicated in the treatment of osteoporosis.
Ovarian Disease	Studies show that high-dose oral contraceptives can prevent functional ovarian cysts. There is early evidence that low-dose pills may have the same health benefit. However, the treatment of already existing ovarian cysts with the use of OCs usually has not proved successful. Of far greater importance is the significant reduction of ovarian cancer already described.
Pain Relief	Analgesics have been studied to analyze whether there is a significant drug interaction with OCs. Acetaminophen and possibly aspirin appear to have their actions modified by the use of OCs; it may be necessary for OC users to take a larger dose of the analgesic.
Pelvic Inflammatory Disease (PID)	The use of oral contraceptives has been shown to reduce the risks of PID, as previously noted. Women who have a history of PID or who have active disease may use the pill.

Pituitary Microadenomas	A number of years ago researchers thought that these tumors of the pituitary gland were produced by the administration of oral contraceptives. However, this is no longer considered the case. Also, the presence of a pituitary microadenoma is not a contraindication to OC use.
Polycystic Ovarian Disease	One of the symptoms of this fairly common endocrine disorder is irregular menses. This particular symptom has been considered to be an indication for the use of the OCs. Menstrual irregularity, acne, hirsutism, and amenorrhea, also parts of this syndrome, are often alleviated to some degree by OC use.
Porphyria	A number of different clinical presentations of this inborn error of metabolism known as porphyria have major systemic symptoms. One form of this disease is known as ovulocytic porphyria. In this instance, the attacks are associated with menstrual periods. Current research indicates that OCs may be of considerable value in protecting against menstrual porphyria.
Postabortion/Postpartum	Oral contraceptives may be started shortly after either a spontaneous or induced abortion. The postpartum use of OCs in both breast-feeding and non-breast-feeding women is covered in detail elsewhere in this chapter. A woman who has delivered a full-term baby should delay OC use for two weeks because of the very small risk of a venous thrombosis. However, with low-dose pills, many women actually start at the time of leaving the hospital. This is also true for progestin-only pills, which are considered the OC drug of choice for women who are going to breast-feed.

Pregnancy	Known or suspected pregnancy is listed as an absolute contraindication to OC administration in the labeling of all oral contraceptives and is classified by the World Health Organization in Category IV. However, it should be mentioned here that many women have attempted to use OCs to induce abortion and that these attempts have been uniformly unsuccessful.
Premenstrual Syndrome (PMS)	Studies have suggested that in up to 30 percent of women, the use of oral contraceptives may help to reduce some of the symptoms associated with PMS. These effects are probably due to the suppression of ovulation.
Rheumatoid Arthritis	For a time, the reduction of the risk of developing rheumatoid arthritis was considered to be among the possible noncontraceptive health benefits of OC use. In recent years, however, there have been questions as to whether or not this is a significant effect, and the studies in this area are highly controversial. At present, the prevailing view is that OC use probably does not prevent rheumatoid arthritis. On the other hand, there is some evidence that OCs may slow the progression of the disease.
Schistosomiasis	Schistosomiasis is an infection caused by blood flukes, parasites that are found in both animals and humans. It is a very common condition in Africa and in Southeast Asia. People who have this disease may use OCs unless there has been severe liver damage in which case OCs are contraindicated.
Seizures	Studies of OC users who have one of the seizure disorders have revealed no impact on either the frequency or the pattern of the attacks. Some of the drugs employed to treat epilepsy produced drug

interactions that lead to a lowering of the estrogen and/or progestin levels sufficient to allow ovulation. The most commonly used anticonvulsants that have been shown to have this effect are phenobarbital and phenytoin; some of the other anticonvulsants are also suspected of decreasing the efficiency of OCs, but these have not been as well studied. For this reason, these women usually are prescribed an OC containing 50 mcg of estrogen.

Sexually Transmitted Diseases

Women who have an active STD or those who give a history of having an infection in the past, as well as women who are at increased risk for the transmission of an STD, should not be prohibited from using OCs. As has been noted elsewhere in this chapter, although there appears to be a lowered risk of acquiring certain bacterial diseases, OCs are not protective against the development of infections with any of the viral STDs.

Sickle Cell Disease

Sickle cell disease is caused by a genetic mutation that results in abnormalities in red blood cells. Several reports published about thirty years ago suggested that there was an association between the use of OCs and the thromboembolic complications that occurred in some women with sickle cell disease. More recent studies have failed to show this association and, at the present time, OC use is not contraindicated for women with this disease. In fact, because women with sickle cell disease have a much higher incidence of complications if they become pregnant, prevention of unwanted pregnancy is a key consideration.

Smoking

The WHO guidelines place smoking in both Category III and Category IV. The first group consists of women who smoke up to twenty cigarettes per day

Smoking (continued)	and are under thirty-five years of age; once women smoke more than that number and are older than thirty-five, OC use is contraindicated. Thus a highly significant risk, Category IV, is only found in these older smokers, particularly if they smoke heavily. The Category III contraindication for younger women is only a relative one inasmuch as the risks of cardiovascular damage are quite low in this age group, even in those who smoke. Someone who has not smoked for a year can be classified as a non-smoker. The very low-dose pills or the minipill may be appropriate in this situation as they have little or no impact on clotting factors, regardless of the age of the woman.
Steroids	The use of steroids as anti-inflammatory agents is not a contraindication to OC use. However, taking the pill may increase the biological effects of the steroid, sometimes necessitating a decrease in the dose.
Stroke	Women who have had a documented stroke should not be considered candidates for OC use.
Surgery	Major surgery, particularly chest and abdominal procedures, is a contraindication to OC use because of the increased risk of thromboembolic complications. When surgery is to be carried out on elective basis for OC users, the pill should be stopped approximately one month prior to surgery and not resumed until about a month afterward. Prolonged immobilization is also a contraindication for the same reason. Anticoagulation has been recommended for women on OCs who have emergency surgery.

Systemic Lupus Erythematosus (SLE) Since SLE can be exacerbated by the use of estrogen, combined pills are usually contraindicated for women with this disease. If the disease has already caused vascular complications, this then becomes an absolute contraindication. On the other hand, it is possible to consider the use of the progestin-only pill in this condition.

Thalassemia Thalassemia is an inherited blood disorder that results in changes in the hemoglobin of the red blood cells. The presence of this disease is not a contraindication to OC use.

Thrombophlebitis Active deep vein thrombosis or a history of this condition, with or without pulmonary embolism, are both absolute contraindications to the use of OCs.

Thyroid Disease There is no reason to deny women who have thyroid disorders use of OCs. This includes those with hyperthyroid and hypothyroid disease states as well as women with simple goiter.

Trophoblastic Disease A history of either benign or malignant gestational trophoblastic disease (tumors arising from a pregnancy) is not a contraindication to OC use.

Tuberculosis (TB) Women with active TB or a history of the disease can use OCs. However, those using rifampin as part of their therapy should be given a 50 mcg OC because of a known drug interaction.

Ulcerative Colitis There is no reason to consider this disease of the lower large bowel a contraindication to the use of the oral contraceptives, as they have not been found to produce any changes in the clinical pattern of this

Ulcerative Colitis (continued)	disorder. Also the effectiveness of the OCs is not diminished because the drugs are absorbed mainly in the upper small bowel.
Unexplained Vaginal Bleeding	A woman who presents with vaginal bleeding typical of the irregular patterns which are quite common among healthy women and who has no other symptoms or signs of significant pelvic disease, should be allowed to use the pill. However, if the bleeding pattern is unexplained, it should be thoroughly investigated before the woman begins using an OC. If abnormal unexplained bleeding occurs during pill use, it is also necessary to evaluate the reason for this symptom, particularly if it persists or if it appears that it might be caused by an infection or a malignancy.
Urinary Tract Infections	The history or presence of a urinary tract infection is not a contraindication to the use of the oral contraceptives.
Uterine Fibroids	In the days of the high-dose OCs, it was noted that preexisting fibroids sometimes grew and on occasion degenerated. These changes were similar to those sometimes seen with pregnancy, under the influence of high hormonal levels. However, with the current use of the low-dose pills, the presence of fibroids is not a contraindication inasmuch as they do not stimulate their growth. In fact, there is early evidence that use of OCs might lower the risk of developing this condition.
Varicose Veins	Superficial varicosities are not a contraindication to OC use. The history or presence of superficial thrombophlebitis is considered to be in the WHO Category II, since the benefits of OC use are felt to

outweigh the risks. On the other hand, deep vein thrombosis and/or thrombophlebitis with or without pulmonary embolization are absolute contraindications.

Weight Gain

Despite the fact that there is a common misperception that the use of oral contraceptives will cause weight gain, this has not been found to be true. Significant increases in weight are usually found only in individuals who have a very poor diet and who fail to carry out sufficient exercise to help to control their weight. Also, it is well known that women tend to put on weight gradually as they age.

Return of Fertility

Most women who have used OCs begin to ovulate again within six weeks of the time that they stop their pills. This is similar to the duration of time seen in women who have delivered a baby, but who are not breast-feeding.

When women stop OC use in order to establish a pregnancy, there may be a one- to three-month delay. About half of this group will be pregnant by three months, and about 90 percent by the end of two years. This is the same rate found in the general population of non-contracepting women and those who have used barrier methods and IUDs. If infertility persists much past one year, a careful medical evaluation is advised.

Women who have the longest delays in establishing a pregnancy are those who are older and who are experiencing a natural decrease in their fertility. A delay is also more common in women who had a history of irregular menses prior to use of the pill, and may be an indication of some underlying gynecologic problem.

If pregnancy occurs with the first ovulation, it is necessary to take into account the fact that their delivery date may be off by two or three weeks because of the delay in the resumption of ovulation.

Women coming off the pill to become pregnant often use a barrier contraceptive for the first month to make the timing of their delivery date more accurate.

Problems in establishing a pregnancy do not relate to the length of time that the pill was taken. Also, studies show that pregnancies immediately following OC use do not result in higher spontaneous abortion rates, nor is there an increase in any other complication of pregnancy.

Fetal Effects

A number of years ago, reports began to appear in the medical literature suggesting that damage was occurring to fetuses conceived while a woman was using oral contraceptives. These included transposition of the great vessels of the heart as well as anomalies known as VAC-TEL (vertebral, anal, cardiac, tracheal, esophageal, and limb) abnormalities. Also a higher incidence of one particular type of abnormal chromosome was reported.

All these reports were a major source of concern for a considerable period of time. However, subsequent and better controlled studies have explained many of these findings and have also failed to confirm any risks of this nature to babies conceived while pill taking was continued. Thus, most of the concerns about fetal abnormalities have been laid to rest with both better analyses of the previously reported studies and with new evaluations of the situation using detailed epidemiological data. Today there is no warning in any of the pill labeling indicating that there is any risk.

In countries such as Sweden, where there is excellent medical surveillance, no increase in congenital anomalies has been found. Also, there has been no higher incidence of perinatal morbidity or mortality, prematurity, or the risk of having a baby with Down's syndrome. In addition, several detailed long-term follow-up studies have been conducted on children who were exposed to OCs in the early months of pregnancy. These have evaluated many things including weight, anemia, intelligence, and general levels of development; no abnormalities have been detected in any of these studies.

In the past, it was suggested that several ovulations be allowed to occur prior to the establishment of a pregnancy because of a perceived risk to the fetus if this was not done. However, no data have ever been found that would substantiate this suggestion. In fact, one study reported a lower incidence of Down's syndrome in infants conceived shortly after their mothers had discontinued the use of OCs. Finally, babies born to previous OC users have been found to be heavier and have lower perinatal death rates. However, this may well be the result of better timing and spacing of pregnancies and better prenatal care.

Myths

There have always been many myths and numerous bits of misinformation about OC use. These have been perpetuated by all types of media, particularly when reporting on the thesis of a research paper that suggests a possible adverse clinical event. Very often media coverage of such papers tends to be very brief; as a result, sometimes very complicated issues are not explored, leaving the reader or viewer with a skewed interpretation. Also, when reporting adverse effects of the oral contraceptives, only rarely do the media include the concept of the risk/benefit ratio in their presentations. Surveys have shown that the impact of an adverse report on a drug or device usually continues for several months and that usage of the product rarely returns to its previous level. For many years the media resisted presenting the noncontraceptive health benefits of OCs, although fortunately this is beginning to change.

The fear most frequently expressed by women concerns the development of breast cancer as a result of OC use; the intensity of the anxiety escalates each time there is a media report of a possible risk. As pointed out earlier in this chapter, fears in this instance are either groundless or vastly overrated. At the same time, the protection against ovarian and uterine cancer is rarely mentioned by the media.

Adolescents have several fears about using OCs. Their biggest fear in this area concerns potential weight gain, although the data do not support this as a proved side effect. In addition, adolescents have greater emotional responses to the publication of "bad news" about the pill, and also react to the development of adverse side effects far more strongly than do older women.

Counseling

As is the case with virtually any medication, the degree of compliance and the chances of continuation depend very heavily on the counseling that a woman receives at the time of the initiation of her therapy. This is particularly true in the case of the oral contraceptives because of the fact that often the information a woman already has may well be incomplete or incorrect. She is likely to have some of the fears already noted, and there may be a number of things in her personal life that make counseling particularly essential.

When a woman elects to use OCs, a number of steps should be taken. First of all, she should be shown a package of the pills that she will be taking and told how they prevent unplanned pregnancy. She should be instructed on when to start her pills; great emphasis must be placed on picking a specific time of day for pill taking, one that fits best into her personal schedule and one that she can remember. She must be told what to do if she misses pills. She must also be made aware of the fact that starting a new cycle of pills late is as serious and potentially more serious than missing individual pills.

The various side effects and their anticipated duration should be gone over very carefully with her as it is essential that she understand these in order to ensure good compliance and continuation. The annoying but nonthreatening side effects that in all likelihood will go away in a short period of time should be discussed. She must be warned of any adverse signs and symptoms that would require immediate medical consultation. She should particularly be made aware of the noncontraceptive health benefits of OCs.

Health practitioners should ask the woman to return in one to two months. By this time, she may have questions about her pill taking, and she may very well have developed some side effects. In both these instances, she will need additional guidance and reassurance if she is to continue with her OC use.

Every OC user should be advised to always have backup methods such as male latex condoms available in the event that she does miss more than one pill and she should know when and how they are to be used. The need for condoms in addition to the OCs is important to assess from the perspective of a woman's new partner(s) or her current partner(s) developing new partners. Condoms should be used under these circumstances for the prevention of STD transmission. Moreover, the OC user should have emergency contraception pills (ECPs) available in the event of a major lapse in her OC use. Finally the outline of her future follow-up care should be laid out at this time.

It is often helpful to accompany verbal counseling with the viewing of an appropriate video. In addition, written material geared to a woman's reading level and in her primary language should be supplied for future review.

Resting

For many years some health-care providers have counseled their patients to take a rest from the use of the pills, sometimes as much as three months out of each year. This subject is mentioned here only in order to vigorously condemn it. There has never been any proof that this type of resting offers any benefit. It does, however, have two major complications. The first is amenorrhea, usually lasting about nine months and ending with an unplanned birth. The second is the redevelopment of the early annoying side effects of pill use which may well occur each time that the oral contraceptives are restarted after an unnecessary rest.

Compliance/Continuation

Compliance and continuation are often hampered when patients become confused due to improper counseling. They frequently do not have appropriate materials that they can read and understand, and, after a time, they become frustrated and decide that it is not worth the effort, particularly if they develop side effects; the result is that they stop using their pills.

Although the failure rate with the use of the oral contraceptives should only be about 1 percent, it has been clear for many years that, due to inconsistencies in actual use, it is often considerably higher. The correct and continued use of OCs is needed in order to achieve a high level of effectiveness. The failure rate, particularly among adolescents, is estimated to be as high as 15 to 20 percent (and sometimes is even higher). This is not due to failure of the pill itself, but to the adolescents' failure to take it properly. Moreover, it is unfortunately quite common for women taking the pill, particularly teenagers, to get distracted by problems such as irregular bleeding or to become anxious because of what they hear about possible adverse OC side effects. Also they may break up with a partner and stop taking the pill, only to resume sexual intercourse at a time when they can become pregnant.

One important recently published study looked at the international impact of incorrect pill taking. It was estimated that if the errors in pill-taking were reduced by only 1 percent a year, this would translate into the prevention of 630,000 unintended pregnancies, nearly 190,000 of which would be in the United States. Another survey showed that only 42 percent of women take their OCs every day. In still another, 16 percent of the subjects who had their pill packages checked at the end of a month were found not to have used all their pills. When evaluating the issue of taking the pill at the same time every day, it was found that more than 80 percent of those surveyed did not do so. Furthermore, even though women in another study were carefully instructed about the use of backup contraception methods, only about a quarter of those who were in a situation where they should have used a backup method actually did so.

Data from several abortion facilities have shown that more than 25 percent of the women asking for a pregnancy termination had been using oral contraceptives during the month in which they became pregnant. Another study showed that only 28 percent of the women interviewed were actually taking their oral contraceptives at the same time every day and did not miss any pills, whereas 27 percent had missed one or more pills during the three months prior to the survey.

Women who fail to continue the OC use do so for a number of well-recognized reasons. One study found that between a quarter and a half of all of the women who started OCs stopped during the first year of use. The main reasons for their discontinuations were found to be the fear of side effects or the actual occurrence of side effects, particularly disturbances of their bleeding patterns, plus a variety of other complaints such as nausea, breast tenderness, and weight gain.

Progestin-Only Oral Contraceptives

For many years OCs containing only a progestin, also called the minipill, have been evaluated. In this type of pill, there is no estrogen as in the combined preparations. Progestin-only pills (POPs) are not commonly used in the United States; currently fewer than 1 percent of OC prescriptions are for this type of pill. Two progestins are used in the minipill—one is norgestrel 75 mcg, and the other is norethindrone 350 mcg. The total amount of progestin in the POP is less than that found in most combined pills; low-dose combination pills usually contain 200 to 300 mcg of norgestrel and between 400 and 1,000 mcg of norethindrone. They must be taken daily.

The minipills have several mechanisms of action. First, they suppress the hormones from the pituitary involved in ovulation, but only in about half of the cycles. Second, all progestins change the cervical mucus; the increased viscosity blocks the passage of sperm into the uterus. Third, POPs interfere with the development of the glands of the endometrium. Finally, there have been some studies suggesting that changes may also occur in the fallopian tubes, decreasing the rate of the flow of eggs through the tubes.

The POPs are statistically somewhat less effective than the combined OCs. However, there is a very clear difference in the need for proper pill taking. Whereas it is important that the combined pills be taken at approximately the same time every day, in the case of the minipill, this is absolutely critical. Blood levels of the progestin reach a maximum about two hours after the pill is taken, and the effects on the cervical mucus are noted at about four hours. The protection offered by POPs begins to diminish after about twenty hours. This makes it essential that the pills be taken at precisely the same time every day; clearly, not following an exact pill-taking regimen will increase the risk of unwanted pregnancy. The minipill has been called the "tea-time pill" since, in most instances, sexual intercourse occurs in the evening; therefore it is usually best to take the pill in the late afternoon or early evening. This will allow time for the maximum protection against sperm penetration of the cervical mucus. In all instances, women should determine the pattern of their sexual activity and take the pill approximately four hours before intercourse is most apt to occur.

If a woman realizes that she has missed a pill, she should take it as soon as she recognizes this fact. She should then resume taking her pills at the same time every day. On the other hand, if three hours have elapsed past the time at which she normally takes her pill, she should take her pill and also use a backup contraception method, most often a male latex condom, for at least the next two days. At the end of forty-eight hours, with the resumption of proper pill-taking, the changes in her cervical mucus should be restored.

The most common side effect with the use of POPs is irregular menstrual bleeding. This may occur as spotting, heavy bleeding, breakthrough bleeding, irregularity in cycle length, or, at different times, all of the above. While none of these is a health hazard to the user, they often can be emotionally distressing and are generally regarded as unpleasant and inconvenient. A WHO study found that during the first three months of POP use, more than half of the women reported frequent bleeding, about one-quarter had prolonged bleeding, about 13 percent had irregular bleeding, and 6 percent developed amenorrhea. At least a quarter of these minipill users discontinued because of their bleeding disturbances. Although with the continued use of the POPs there is a general tendency to return to a more normal pattern of bleeding, it rarely becomes totally predictable.

The minipill is very safe. There are certain advantages to having a preparation available that does not contain any estrogen for those women who are unable for medical reasons to use estrogen or those who have adverse estrogen side effects. There are also specific clinical situations, such as hypertension, a history of blood clots, vascular migraine headaches, cigarette smokers who are over the age of thirty-five, and breast-feeding women, which are frequently considered to be indications for use of the minipill. The major use of the POPs at the present time is during breast-feeding. Women who are giving supplementary formulas to their babies should begin the minipill about three weeks after delivery. Those who are breast-feeding exclusively can wait until about six weeks after giving birth.

It has generally been considered that the use of POPs is associated with a slightly higher risk for ectopic pregnancy. However, there is considerable protection, even in this instance, the ectopic pregnancy rate of POP users actually being three times lower than that found in the general population.

Multiple studies have shown that the minipill produces very little effect on lipid and carbohydrate metabolism and coagulation factors. It does not increase blood pressure, nor does it cause increased rates of cardiovascular disease.

As yet there is very little information, because of the minimal use of this type of pill, as to whether or not they have the same noncontraceptive health benefits as the combined pills, particularly the prevention of ovarian and uterine cancer. Also very little is known about the possible risk of cervical and breast cancer among women using the POPs; however, the limited data that do exist do not suggest that there is an increased incidence of either disease.

Emergency Contraception

Emergency contraception (EC), previously called the morning-after pill and also known as post-coital contraception and interception, has been used for many years. However, *emergency contraception* is now the preferred term because it makes clear the fact that this is not a regular form of contraception, but is to be used only in cases of emergency. Furthermore, the term *morning-after pill* implied that the morning after the night before was the time to use the medication; however, it is now well known that it can be taken any time for up to seventy-two hours after unprotected sex, and some researchers believe that this period of time could be extended to four or five days, similar to the use of an IUD for this indication, but without its long-term protection.

It was originally believed that the ECPs acted directly on the endometrium, interfering with implantation by disturbing the normal hormonal pattern that is essential for the successful development of a pregnancy. However, newer evidence suggests it may be mainly due to either a suppression of or a delay in ovulation. Other possible mechanisms of action include a decrease in the viability of sperm, changes in sperm transport because of alterations in tubal activity, or the blocking of fertilization.

Although at first EC was prescribed mainly for rape victims, it gradually began to enjoy wide usefulness for the general population. It is now being given not only to women who have had unprotected sexual intercourse but also to those in situations such as condom breakage or dislodgement of a diaphragm or cervical cap during coitus, in which pregnancy is a possibility.

The first agent to be used for EC was an estrogen, diethylstilbestrol (DES). It was given in 25 mg doses twice a day for five days after unprotected midcycle intercourse. It was recommended that it be started within the first twelve to twenty-four hours after exposure, but not used after forty-eight hours. Although this particular regimen was quite effective, it had a high incidence of nausea, vomiting, abnormal bleeding, and breast tenderness. Also, it was later reported that the drug could possibly cause damage to female fetuses if a pregnancy continued. Therefore, research continued, attempting to find other hormonal agents that would prevent pregnancy as effectively as DES had, but without its adverse side effects.

A number of different hormonal preparations have been assessed as potential ECPs. Most of the current methods of EC contain both an estrogen and a progestin. In the mid-1960s and early 1970s, many studies were carried out looking for the best products for this indication. The first most widely known, frequently used, and carefully studied approach was the Yuzpe method, named for the Canadian physician who developed it, Dr. Albert Yuzpe. This regimen consists of 0.1 mg of ethinyl estradiol and 1.0 mg of norgestrel. It is taken within three days after unprotected intercourse and then repeated twelve hours later. This form of EC has been available in Europe since 1984.

At the present time, twenty different EC techniques are available, using the currently approved oral contraceptives. The number and administration of each OC is now well established for most of the combined contraceptives, but the correct use of these pills, which are quite different in appearance, can be very difficult and confusing. Progestin-only pills could be used; however, it would take a total of forty tablets given over a twelve-hour span to achieve adequate pregnancy protection.

About 30 to 50 percent of the women using the Yuzpe regimen develop nausea; vomiting occurs in about 20 percent. In attempts to reduce these side effects, it has been recommended that antiemetic medications be taken about an hour before the first dose is administered. Meclizine reduces nausea in from 64 percent to 47 percent of women; also the symptoms are less severe. However, women given Meclizine had a considerably higher rate of drowsiness—twice that of the control group. Furthermore, once women develop nausea and vomiting, antiemetics do very little good. If vomiting occurs, as is often the case within an hour of taking the medication, the pills must be retaken. In addition, breast tenderness has also been reported in almost half of women using the Yuzpe regimen.

Another approach to EC, used in other countries for almost twenty years, is to administer 0.75 mg of levonorgestrel in a single dose within seventy-two hours of unprotected intercourse and repeat in twelve hours. This regimen was approved for EC use by the FDA in July 1999.

After early studies indicated that the use of levonorgestrel might have certain advantages over the Yuzpe method, the WHO set up a large double-blind randomized trial in twenty-one centers in Australia, Canada, China, India, New Zealand, Nigeria, Sweden, the United Kingdom, and the United States. Almost two thousand women were followed in the study, half of them being placed on the standard Yuzpe regimen, the other half being given levonorgestrel alone. In this trial, almost half of the women were given their medication within twenty-four hours of unprotected intercourse, and 80 percent were treated within forty-eight hours. The results of this study showed that the levonorgestrel used alone had a higher rate of success in preventing pregnancy—85 percent as compared to what would have been anticipated with no treatment. Comparable data using the Yuzpe method showed only a 57 percent rate of protection.

What was also of great importance was the observation that the levonorgestrel group had considerably fewer side effects. Nausea and vomiting were seen in both groups, but nausea occurred in 23 percent of the levonorgestrel group and 51 percent of the Yuzpe group. Vomiting occurred in only 6 percent of the levonorgestrel group as compared with 19 percent for the Yuzpe method. The levonorgestrel group also had significantly lower rates of dizziness, fatigue, headaches, breast tenderness, and irregular bleeding.

Earlier reports had suggested that the effectiveness of emergency contraception was very similar for all time periods if the medication was taken within the first seventy-two hours after exposure. However, increasing amounts of data made it clear that this was not the case; the earlier the treatment was given, the higher was the degree of success.

The only contraindication to the use of ECPs is a documented pregnancy. It also needs to be emphasized that the use of this approach will not induce an abortion; many women have tried this without success. If there is a treatment failure and the pregnancy continues, there is no evidence that any adverse effects will be found due to the action of the hormones on a developing fetus.

It is both ironic and instructive that studies carried out at abortion clinics have shown that between 50 and 60 percent of the women that they saw would have been suitable for the use of EC and would have used it if they had known it was available. The National Academy of Sciences has estimated that one half of the 6.3 million pregnancies occurring in the United States each year are unintended and half of these are the result of contraceptive failures. Use of ECPs could prevent 1.7 million of these unplanned pregnancies and could reduce the number of abortions from 1.5 million to 800,000.

One study focused on how well EC would be used under two different sets of conditions. In the first instance, women were only given information about the technique, and in the second group women were given exactly the same information but were also provided with a package of pills. It was found that giving supplies increased the use of EC, but that information alone did not.

Two new commercial products have been developed and approved by the FDA. The first, known as PREVEN™, was approved on September 1, 1998. It contains four pills, each a combination of 50 mcg ethinyl estradiol and 0.25 mg of levonorgestrel. Two pills are taken within seventy-two hours of unprotected intercourse and the other two twelve hours later.

On July 28, 1999, the FDA approved the use of the levonorgestrel regimen, two tablets of 0.75 mg of levonorgestrel, one to be taken immediately after unprotected sex and the other twelve hours later. This is being marketed under the trade name Plan B™. It is currently available by prescription through nonprofit groups such as Planned Parenthood and from clinicians who have been registered with the Emergency Contraception Hotline (1-888-NOT-2-LATE). The number of distribution channels is increasing, and ECPs are gradually becoming more widely used.

Major efforts are now under way to increase the availability of these two FDA-approved products. Many women are unaware of this form of protection against unwanted pregnancy. Emergency contraception is now prescribed by a clinician over the telephone after careful questioning indicates no likelihood of a preexisting pregnancy. Recognizing that this approach to preventing unwanted births was being badly underutilized, pharmacists in 111 drug stores in Washington state set up a pilot study. They developed a collaborative agreement under which women could receive their ECPs directly from a pharmacist. The program was extremely successful, and it is possible that this approach may pave the way for similar methods in other states where there is no legal reason not to do so. The distribution of ECPs through pharmacies has been well accepted by women. It has the clear advantage of reducing the amount of time that elapses before starting the pills, which results in a higher level of effectiveness. It avoids the delays often experienced by women in getting an appointment with their health-care provider or obtaining medication at a time when no medical facilities are open.

In contrast, a striking example of the many problems American women face when trying to control their fertility is the outright refusal of the world's largest retailer, under pressure from antichoice groups, to allow its 2,428 pharmacies to fill doctors' prescriptions for PREVEN™. A company spokesperson has said that never before has it refused to sell any other prescription. Such a move will have its greatest impact in small towns where the smaller local drug stores have been driven out of business. Moreover, individual pharmacists and a 1,500-member pharmacy group have also refused to provide ECPs to their customers. Despite these setbacks, more and more women are learning about EC and are beginning to ask their doctors for this form of help in preventing unwanted pregnancies.

Efforts are being made to move ECPs to OTC status. A citizen's petition was submitted to the FDA in February 2001 by more than 70 organizations, notably including the American Public Health Association (APHA). The petition states that ECPs may be safely and correctly used without professional intervention. The FDA will review the material provided in the petition and make a ruling in the near future.

A number of laws have been passed by Congress over the years defining the situations under which a drug can be sold OTC. Products are to remain on prescription when it is deemed necessary to do so in order to protect the public health. However, a drug is to be made available OTC if the condition to be treated can be diagnosed by a consumer, if it is safe and effective for self-administration, and if it is labeled in language understandable by the average consumer. Those groups urging a move to make these products available without a prescription point out that in addition to meeting the above criteria, ECPs are not dangerous or addictive, they are not toxic to the user or harmful to a developing fetus, and they do not require medical intervention for proper use. Moreover, making these agents available OTC would permit early and easy access, thus reducing the number of unplanned pregnancies and induced abortions. France, Norway, and Great Britain have already instituted OTC procedures.

Multiple attempts have been undertaken to increase the availability and use of ECPs. Prescriptions by telephone and publications of 800 numbers are both being found to be highly effective. Equally and in some instances even more effective is the advance provision of ECPs providing immediate access in case of an emergency, an approach currently being used in the United States, Scotland, and Ghana.

Another new approach, called the Emergency Contraceptive Connection, was started on August 2, 2000, by Planned Parenthood of Georgia, using its secure Internet website. A woman can fill out an application stating where she can be reached and the name of her pharmacy, and then complete a questionnaire, including her medical history, the protocol for which was developed by physicians. This information is then reviewed by a nurse practitioner. If the caller is found to be an appropriate candidate, her prescription is called in and she can go to her pharmacy and get her medication. She can request one of the two commercial products or—for reasons of confidentiality—get one of the OCs with appropriate instructions. This program has been very successful and is being duplicated in other areas of the country with variations dictated by local laws.

Future Trends

In recent years the proportion of women using multiphasic versus monophasic OCs has been reversed. Currently, monophasic pills account for almost 60 percent of the market; multiphasic pills— almost all of them triphasic pills—account for nearly all of the rest. Another change that has occurred has been the increase in the utilization of the 20 mcg pills, which rose by 143 percent between 1996 and 1998, going from 2.3 million to 5.6 million.

The age of the individuals using OCs has also changed during this time period. In 1996, women over the age of forty accounted for almost half of the consumption of the 20 mcg pills. This figure dropped to 28 percent by 1998. Women ages twenty to thirty-nine now are using nearly 60 percent of all 20 mcg pills. This is an increase from 44 percent two years ago. In addition, the numbers of adolescents and teens using the 20 mcg pills has doubled since 1996.

The 20 mcg estrogen pills represent a major decline in dosage over the last forty years. Whether this amount can be decreased still further remains unclear but research is ongoing. It is clear that there has got to be a point at which further lowering of the dose will produce an increase in failures, and possibly an increase in the number and severity of adverse side effects.

New progestins continue to be explored. For example, drospirenon, which will be marketed as Yasmin™, was approved by the FDA in May 2001. Studies have suggested that this progestin is quite similar to naturally occurring progesterone. It has been found to have less effect on fluid retention, leading to stable or possibly slightly lowered body weights. It appears to have a beneficial effect on the symptoms of PMS; improvements in skin conditions have also been noted, as well as an increase in the feeling of well-being. Hopefully this and other future products that produce fewer adverse side effects will result in better compliance and continuation rates.

Summary

Aside from purely medical considerations, the emergence of the pill has had multiple impacts on women and on their place in society. It has allowed them to enjoy their sexual lives without the constant fear of unwanted pregnancies. It has changed their perceptions of themselves in relation to their own lives and those of their families. It has altered their attitudes toward their sexual behavior and toward the timing and extent of their childbearing. Finally, it has introduced a new dimension into their interpersonal relationships with their husbands and their sexual partners.

3

Contraceptive Implants

LABORATORY RESEARCH INTO the development of subdermal contra-ceptive implants was undertaken in 1966. One implant, known today as Norplant, has been used in clinical trials since 1975. These trials have been carried out in forty-six countries and have involved fifty-five thousand women. The implant is currently approved for use in more than twenty countries, and more than six million women have used it worldwide.

The idea for this form of contraception stemmed from the notion that it might be possible to put chemicals into silastic tubing that would allow them to come out gradually, depending on the type of material used, over a considerable period of time. Several different progestins were studied. Some of these were found to be effective for only one year, while others were found not to be practical because it was impossible to get a level high enough to be contraceptive. Finally, levonorgestrel became the drug of choice. The reasoning behind this decision was twofold. First, it was possible to get sufficient progestin into the silastic tubing to last for five years. Second, this particular agent was well known because it had been used as part of combined oral contraceptives for many years.

Studies on the Norplant System were undertaken by the Popula-tion Council in New York and were carried out in many countries over a period of thirty years. Data from these trials helped to win

FDA approval in December 1990. Manufacturing and distribution began in 1991. Norplant was actually the first major new contraceptive agent to be developed and introduced in the United States in the 1990s. To date, more than 1 million American women have had the Norplant System inserted.

Early in the use of the Norplant System, a number of physicians and other health-care providers were trained in the proper insertion and removal techniques; this training was essential for the proper use of this product. In response to concerns on the part of the Norplant manufacturer that financially disadvantaged women might not have access to this contraceptive method, it established The Norplant Foundation, which provided money for clinicians trained and authorized to do insertions and removals for financially disadvantaged eligible women.

The currently available subdermal implant consists of six flexible closed capsules of silicone rubber; each is 34.0 mm long and 2.4 mm in diameter and contains 36 mg of levonorgestrel. The capsules are placed just beneath the skin in a spoke shape. They provide a constant slow release of levonorgestrel starting with 80 mg a day, going to 50 mg at nine to twelve months, and blood levels of 30 to 35 mg are maintained for at least five years. Some investigators now believe that the period of effectiveness may actually be as long as seven years.

Levonorgestrel is absorbed into the systemic circulation at a mean rate of 350 pg/mL during these five years of use. The daily dose is similar to that of the minipill and is about one-fourth to one-third of that of the combined OCs. Contraceptive levels are reached within a day following implantation and return to normal within ninety-six hours of removal.

The insertion should be carried out within five to seven days after the start of a normal menstrual period to avoid administration during an early and unrecognized pregnancy. Provided that the technician is skilled, the insertion is usually quite easy. The removal may be more difficult, particularly if the capsules were not put in properly or were placed too deep, in which case it may take up to half an hour or more. When any foreign body is inserted, a fibrous sheath is formed around it; this is true regardless of the nature of the material. When the sheaths around the Norplant are nicked during the removal process, the implants usually slide out quite easily. The implants can be removed at any time. Once the Norplant System is out, fertility returns very promptly to the level the woman had prior to the insertion. This return is unrelated to the amount of time the woman has worn her Norplant. Eighty percent of women begin to ovulate in three weeks and almost all start within seven weeks after removal. In one study, 86 percent of women trying to conceive did so within one year. This is the same rate as is seen following the use of OCs, IUDs, or no method at all.

The Norplant has been shown to exert its protection against pregnancy in several ways. First, it blocks ovulation in less than half of the users. A second major mechanism of action is thickening of the cervical mucus, caused by the progestin. This interferes with the passage of sperm up through the cervix into the uterus and the tubes. Finally, it also suppresses endometrial development.

Norplant is highly effective, pregnancy rates being less than 1 percent. Many studies have shown no pregnancies at all in the first year of use. Over the next four years, rates have been 0.2 percent, 0.9 percent, 0.5 percent, and 1.1 percent respectively. Overall, the failure rate is estimated to be about 0.2 percent.

Earlier studies on the Norplant System showed that women who weighed more than 78 kg had higher pregnancy rates than those who weighed less than 50 kg. For a time, it was believed that heavier women were not good candidates for the use of Norplant. The discrepancy was cleared up with continued research; the earlier implants were made of a dense tubing material which limited the release of the progestin. When this was identified as the problem, the implants were then made of less dense material; this allowed a more consistent and sustained release of the levonorgestrel. Following the move to the new tubing, the pregnancy rates among heavier women very closely approximated those obtained in lighter women.

Insertions

It is essential that the implants be properly inserted. If the insertion is faulty, the removal process can be very difficult. Prior to the insertion of the implants, women are given a local anesthetic and, in most instances, the insertions are not painful. After cleaning the skin with an antiseptic, the implants are placed in the upper inner nondominant arm approximately 8 to 10 cm above the elbow crease, where they are less apt to be visible. They are placed just below and parallel to the skin in a fanlike arrangement with a 75-degree arc, a distance of 5 mm apart at the base.

When done by a physician or a nurse practitioner with proper training and experience, insertions take approximately five to ten minutes. Often an ice pack is placed over the injection site for twenty to thirty minutes and a pressure dressing is applied for the first two days to reduce the chance of swelling. The area where the implants were inserted may be slightly tender for up to one week, and bruising may be noted for approximately the same length of time. In less than 1 percent of cases, there may be infection, bleeding, or expulsion.

Removals

The removal process almost always takes more time than the insertion. If the implants were properly inserted, removal is usually a simple procedure lasting somewhere between ten and forty minutes.

Most removals are carried out under a local anesthetic injected under the tips of the rods. The majority of removals cause little or no discomfort. Removals that take longer and may be painful are usually related to poor insertion, poor positioning of the rods, or breaking of the rods. If the rods were placed too deeply below the skin, they may become embedded in the tissues of the arm.

Removals are usually carried out by making a small (3.0 to 5.0 mm) incision at the tips of the rods. Each rod is pushed gently toward the incision; the tip is then grasped either with an instrument or the fingers, the fibrous sheath is opened, and the rod is removed. A number of different removal techniques have been developed over the years in attempts to find the quickest and least traumatic approach. In addition, a number of special instruments have been designed to facilitate removals.

Side Effects

The most common side effects noted by many women early in the use of their subdermal implants are changes in their bleeding patterns. Most women have a temporary change in the pattern and amount of bleeding, their menses often becoming quite irregular; a few actually stop having periods. These changes occur predominantly in the first year of use. Thereafter, the majority of women return to a cycle similar to the one that they had prior to the insertion. The most common irregularities include episodes of spotting and prolonged bleeding and the total number of days of bleeding often increases. However, it has been found that the overall blood loss is actually often less than the menstrual period blood loss measured prior to insertion. Following hemoglobin levels in a number of women showed that, in general, the levels increased more frequently than they decreased. Other side effects that have been reported include nausea, headaches, nervousness, dizziness, weight gain, and acne.

Women have had several concerns about implants. The most commonly reported fear is that the implants, since they contain a hormone, may cause cancer at the site of insertion or elsewhere, particularly the breast. There is no evidence that this has ever occurred. A second concern is that they will be left with a big scar. Actually, the implant scars are usually only about a quarter of an inch long, when implants are properly placed and removed. The incisions do not require sutures, and the ultimate scarring is usually minimal. Another concern that some women have is that the implants will move around. This also has not been proved to be true. Rarely, the implants shift slightly after the insertion, but usually less than one inch. Finally, women have worried that the implants will be visible. In the majority of instances, this occurs only in very thin women.

Advantages

The primary advantage of the subdermal implants is their high level of effectiveness. A second advantage is that fertility returns to its previous level very soon after the rods have been taken out, allowing a woman to plan the timing of her next pregnancy. A third advantage is that this technique does not depend on a woman's remembering to use her contraceptive daily or with each act of intercourse. It is not necessary to purchase contraceptive products. Implants do not require cleaning or storage as do some of the barrier techniques. Fourth, this is a safe method; no serious side effects have ever been reported. Fifth, Norplant can be inserted immediately after delivery of a baby; it may be used safely and effectively by women who wish to breast-feed.

Disadvantages

Norplant use requires two surgical procedures, one for insertion and one for removal. While these are usually uneventful, the idea of any surgery is a problem for some women. If left in place for several years, the Norplant System is quite cost-effective but if removed early, it is quite expensive. The primary problems, as noted, are the development of abnormal bleeding patterns and the fact that the rods may be visible in very thin women.

Continuation Rates

Studies have shown that women who choose the subdermal implants continue to use them at a higher rate than they do other methods such as the OCs and barriers; about 90 percent continue for more than one year of use. This is a higher figure than is found with almost all other contraceptive methods. In addition, several studies have shown that continuation rates are much higher among teenage Norplant users than for those choosing OCs, leading to much lower one-year pregnancy rates.

Candidates for Use

Several factors make Norplant a good choice for certain groups of women. Primarily, these are individuals who do not want to have a baby for several more years (if ever), and who are anxious to have a high level of protection against unplanned pregnancy. Often this includes women who have thought about being sterilized but are not willing at that point in their lives to have a procedure that will, to all intents and purposes, prevent all future pregnancies.

There may be medical reasons for women not to use other forms of contraception, especially those containing estrogen where the risk of blood clots is a concern. Where lower progestin doses are desired, the Norplant System may be selected because it contains less hormone than is found in OCs and injectables. Finally, individuals who comply poorly with methods that require daily attention (or methods that are only effective if used with every act of sexual intercourse) are particularly good candidates.

Counseling

As in the case of any medical treatment, the best results come when careful counseling is carried out prior to the institution of therapy. This is particularly true in the case of the subdermal implants. Potential users should be shown what the implants look like. They should understand the insertion process and the procedure for removal. Further, they must be reassured that the rods will not migrate from the insertion site, and will not break if subjected to trauma. It is particularly important in this instance to discuss the fact that, particularly in the first year of use, menstrual pattern abnormalities are to be expected. If a woman is properly informed about the occurrence of these irregularities it will, in most instances, serve to keep her from being overly anxious if and when they do occur. It is also important that she know that she will probably revert to a normal menstrual pattern after about one year of use of her Norplant. It is well documented that bleeding irregularities in most cases will be well tolerated if proper counseling has been carried out.

An important part of counseling women about using the implants is to make sure that they understand that the implants will not protect them against the transmission of STDs or HIV/AIDS. If, in the initial taking of a woman's history, it is found that she is at risk for these diseases, it is critical that she recognize that she will have no protection and that she ought to use condoms in addition to her Norplant. Also she must be aware that she can become pregnant as soon as the implants are removed.

The level of usage of the Norplant System is lower today than it was previously estimated that it would be. Several surveys have shown a number of reasons for this unanticipated outcome. Many women, more than 25 percent, reported being happy with their current method. An increasing number of women in the various surveys expressed fears about using Norplant, undoubtedly the result of negative media publicity about problems with the method itself and also the allegations of coercive use in certain, primarily disadvantaged, women. Many respondents said that they either did not know about Norplant, or that they did not know enough to make it a good option. Finally, a second long-term progestin-only injectable agent, Depo-Provera™ became available which may have decreased the number of women who otherwise might have elected to use the implants.

Some surveys show that the failure to select the Norplant System is most often based on lack of knowledge about the method coupled with unreasonable fears about its use. Therefore, public education could be of great value in increasing acceptance—a recommendation common to all contraceptive methods.

Litigation

Norplant became the object of considerable legal action in the early 1990s. Numerous lawsuits were filed soon after adverse media presentations, most notably a very inflammatory, grossly distorted, and damaging television show on the implants, which aired on *Face to Face with Connie Chung*. Of interest is the fact that another of her programs, equally erroneous, was a key factor in stimulating a feeding frenzy by the plaintiffs' attorneys during the silicone gel-filled breast implant disaster. This ended in a $4 billion settlement to cover several class-action and thousands of individual lawsuits against the implant manufacturers, despite the fact that there was no scientific evidence to support the charges being made. As a result, the Dow Corning Corporation ultimately had to file for Chapter 11 bankruptcy.

It was claimed that Norplant was causing the same patterns of autoimmune disease that had been alleged to be caused by the silicone breast implants. The culprit, these allegations claimed, was a silicone coating on the Norplant rods. It was soon noted that the litigation in these cases followed very closely that seen with the breast implants; often the Norplant lawsuits were filed by the same attorneys citing the same complaints. In fact, a number of the suits filed in different states on the same day contained identical typographical errors. Moreover, many of the same medical "experts" were involved in each of the Norplant lawsuits, as were a number of laboratories making considerable profits from diagnosing what they called silicone-related diseases.

Having learned a few things from the breast implant litigation, this time the plantiffs' attorneys met in Houston in 1995 to map out an integrated plan of attack on Norplant. One speaker even claimed that a woman had died when a rod had migrated to her heart and killed her.

It is critical to note that numerous epidemiological studies carried out in the United States and other countries have not documented any of the adverse effects claimed to result from the use of the silicone breast implants, nor has any serious damage been found in the case of the subdermal implants. However, Norplants were sometimes put in and removed by individuals who had not received sufficient training or who had not carried out the insertion and removal procedures properly. Thus, there were indeed some local complications, and lawsuits claiming injury to arms were legitimate. Because of the rising tide of concern and litigation, the FDA in 1995 did an extensive review of the safety of Norplant. It issued a report on August 17, 1995, stating that no basis had been found as the result of this inquiry to suggest that the implants were not safe and effective when used as directed. It cited data from adverse reaction reports and postmarketing surveillance studies. In addition, the World Health Organization, the American Society for Reproductive Medicine, and a number of other medical groups publicly supported the continued use of Norplant. These organizations expressed their fears that this valuable contraceptive option might be permanently lost.

The utilization of the subdermal implants dropped abruptly in the United States as the result of the adverse media reports and the numerous lawsuits. Sales dropped from eight hundred a day to about sixty.

Medical facilities began to report that removal rates had gone up sharply while insertion rates had dropped considerably. During this same period of time, a survey conducted by the Population Council did not find any lawsuits in the forty-four other countries where Norplant was being used. In 1999, use of the product was actually discontinued in the United Kingdom, reportedly for the same fears of frivolous litigation. In the United States, about fourteen thousand claims were dismissed. The Norplant manufacturer, in August of that year, decided to settle the remaining 36,000 claims. The company recognized that the expense involved in defending all of these lawsuits, even if they were to win the majority of them, was too great. Use of the Norplant is starting to gradually resume, but its eventual role in the overall American contraceptive picture remains uncertain.

Future Implants

Research has been underway for some years attempting to reduce the number of rods that are required for protection against pregnancy. Currently systems utilizing one and two rods have been and are being developed. One of these, known as Norplant II consists of two rods, each 44 mm long and 2.4 mm in diameter, with a core containing 75 mg of leveonorgestrel covered by silicone rubber tubing. It has been shown to have approximately the same pregnancy rates, side effects, and effectiveness as the original six-rod system. It can also be used for five years. Removal is easier and quicker; often health professionals can extract the rods without using instruments. The average removal time is reported at less than sixteen minutes. However, although this new approach has received preliminary FDA approval, there is still a fear that this improved product may never be brought to market in the United States because of potential litigation.

Another implant known as Implanon™ has been studied for several years and FDA approval is currently being sought. It is a single rod, 40 mm long and 2 mm in diameter, which contains 60 mg of crystalline 3-keto-desogestrel in a core of ethinyl vinyl acetate. It behaves much like Norplant and is effective for two to three years. It was approved for three years of use in the United Kingdom in November 1999. A second single rod implant known as Uniplant™ is also being studied. It is 4 mm long and made of silastic tubing. It contains 38 mg of nomegestrol acetate, releasing 100 mcg a day for one year.

A biodegradable implant known as Capronor™ is also currently being evaluated. It is a single capsule made of a polymer, E-caprolactone, and is being tested in two different sizes. One is 2.5 mm long and contains 16 mg of levonorgestrel; the other is 4 mm long and contains 26 mg; both are 0.24 cm in diameter. Since the hormone is released from the polymer ten times faster than from Norplant, it can be smaller in size. The capsules remain intact for twelve months during which time they can be removed if necessary; however, after one year they begin to disintegrate. Women using the smaller capsules usually continue to ovulate; about half using the larger capsules do not, slightly more than with Norplant. Pregnancy rates are being studied but since the larger capsules produce about the same blood levels as the Norplant System, it probably will prove to have equivalent effectiveness rates.

4

Injectable Contraceptives

AN INJECTABLE CONTRACEPTIVE, Depo-Provera™ (DMPA, depot medroxyprogesterone acetate)—also known as the "shot"—like the implant, was used in other countries for many years before getting FDA approval in the United States. It is a long-term method; it is highly effective when given by injection once every three months. Much of what we know about the use of this agent comes from decades of study in a number of countries, particularly Thailand and Mexico where it has been extremely popular and the method of choice for many women.

Depo-Provera has had a lengthy, controversial, and highly politicized history in the United States, and the road to approval was long and tortuous. The first application to the FDA for use as a contraceptive came in 1967, submitted by its manufacturer, the Upjohn Company. DMPA had already been approved since the 1950s for the treatment of uterine and kidney cancers, where it was given in very high doses. It had also been used quite successfully as a form of treatment for endometriosis. In addition, it had been given in attempts to prevent threatened and habitual abortions, but it was found to have little or no value in these cases.

Although DMPA had previously been approved as a contraceptive in more than ninety countries and had been used since the mid-1960s by more than thirty million women, the FDA failed at this time to give its approval. Despite this, since it was available for other indications and was well known in medical circles to be an excellent contraceptive, it was given to thousands of women by their doctors.

The prolonged and repeated refusal of the FDA to approve Depo-Provera as a contraceptive agent has been widely recognized to be a political, not a scientific, decision. One major reason given for its earlier disapprovals was the development, reported in 1972, of breast tumors in beagle dogs that had been selected by the FDA to be used as test animals. Beagles have been known for many years to have high spontaneous rates of both benign and malignant breast tumors. They develop these lesions with all progestins, including natural progesterone, the hormone made by normally ovulating women. Moreover, in these trials, the animals that were studied were given twenty-five times the human contraceptive dose.

The well-documented metabolic changes and the responses of female beagle dogs to progestins are markedly different from those observed in the human female. In contrast to the progressive thinning of the endometrium noted in women, the endometrium of the beagle is overstimulated by the administration of progestins, often leading to uterine infections and death. In recognition of this fact, the FDA at one time even recommended that the dogs have hysterectomies to allow continued observations of other possible adverse effects of DMPA administration. In the 1980s, the World Health Organization, the British and other regulatory agencies, and a number of scientific groups stated that beagle dogs were inappropriate test animals for all steroid hormones and recommended that their use be discontinued. However, it was not until 1992 that the FDA stopped requiring testing in these animals.

Another reason given for the continued disapproval by the FDA was the development of endometrial cancers reported in 1978 in two of ten rhesus monkeys who had been given fifty times the human dose of DMPA in a ten-year study. No cancers were found in twenty monkeys given other doses or in seven control animals. These tumors were found in an epithelial plaque, a type of tissue not found in the uterus of the human female. In addition, this particular tumor had also been observed in two untreated animals, one of which was a control in an IUD study and the other a control in an OC trial. As in the case of the beagle dogs, the required studies on the monkeys have now also finally been rescinded by the FDA.

Even more importantly, there was no epidemiological evidence for an increased risk of endometrial cancer in the human female despite the widespread use of Depo-Provera over a period of many years. In addition, DMPA had long been used successfully in the treatment of women with endometrial cancer, even those in whom the tumor had spread beyond the uterus to other parts of the body. Finally, the protection against this disease seen with the use of combined OCs has now been found also with DMPA; in both instances it has been shown to be due to the action of the progestin.

Of considerable interest in this regard are data gathered from the northern province of Chiang Mai in Thailand. DMPA has been used extensively in that area since the late 1960s; it is estimated that more than 100,000 women selected this method of contraception, and that more than 1,000 women used it in excess of ten years. It was reported at an international forum on DMPA and endometrial cancer that 25 percent of women between the ages of fifteen and forty-four in Chiang Mai were Depo-Provera users. Reviews of hospital records in that area indicated no increase in the incidence of endometrial cancer. Moreover, when women who had developed this disease were traced, no DMPA use was identified.

Data from the animal studies, plus the changes in menstrual patterns and the delayed return of fertility—both of which will subsequently be described—were used by the opponents of Depo-Provera very successfully in helping to block its approval as a contraceptive. Many studies had shown that there was a high incidence of bleeding abnormalities, particularly early in the use of DMPA. Also there was usually a delay of up to a year before ovulation started again and pregnancy could occur. This delay was widely and incorrectly referred to as sterility, with the implication that it was permanent.

In 1973, the FDA's advisory panel unanimously recommended approval of DMPA for a limited patient group. However, the impact of 1974 congressional hearings on Depo-Provera combined with the widespread and well-organized opposition, both of which resulted in extremely adverse media coverage, led to the FDA's putting its approval on hold. The opposition came from certain women's health groups and consumer groups who claimed that DMPA was unsafe and also from religious conservatives who were trying to block the use of all methods of birth control. In 1975, the FDA's advisory panel once again unanimously recommended approval for a limited group, but once again its advice was overruled.

Finally, three years later, in 1978, the FDA formally denied approval of DMPA for use as a contraceptive, claiming a concern about the drug's safety. It stated that it based its decision on a number of considerations such as the beagle dog data and the possibility of producing congenital abnormalities in fetuses in the event of failure, since the drug had such a prolonged duration of action. It also said that the frequent bleeding abnormalities found with the use of Depo-Provera might lead to the use of estrogen; this would impose an additional risk to women and would eliminate the advantages of a progestin-only method. The FDA response further cited the availability of "safer" contraceptive options and stated that there was "no demonstrated need" for DMPA in the United States. Finally, it expressed serious reservations about the ability of the Upjohn Company to carry out the proposed postmarketing studies the company had planned to look for the possible occurrence of cancer in DMPA users.

This decision was appealed by Upjohn and two years later the FDA, in an unusual move, appointed a Public Board of Inquiry. This group met in 1984, and after several days of testimony from researchers, health-care providers, medical organizations, and the general public ruled—to the great surprise and dismay of many scientists—that the available safety data were insufficient for FDA approval.

Meanwhile, in 1979, the World Health Organization had started large-scale studies looking at DMPA and the incidence of cancer. Their results, which were published in 1991, indicated no overall increase in the risk of cancer in Depo-Provera users. In response to these studies and other epidemiological data that also showed no cancer risk, in April 1992 the FDA invited the Upjohn Company to submit a new application for the approval of DMPA as a contraceptive.

Finally, on June 19, 1992, the FDA's Advisory Committee on Fertility and Maternal Health again unanimously recommended its approval. This decision followed extensive testimony by medical experts, particularly those from WHO. Scientific groups, researchers, the manufacturer, and members of the public also made presentations.

On October 29, 1992, DMPA was at last approved as there was no evidence that it was unsafe and led to cancers or other major health problems, and there was a great deal of evidence of its value as a contraceptive option for many women.

The United States was the ninety-second country to approve the use of DMPA as a contraceptive. It remained unapproved in Canada and New Zealand at that time, both countries having experienced the same attacks and media frenzy—often by the same people using the same techniques—that had delayed approval in the United States for twenty-five years.

DMPA acts primarily on the two areas of the brain, the hypothalamus and the pituitary, that control the cyclic release of the hormones that are responsible for the induction of ovulation. When their production is suppressed by the use of DMPA, the development and release of eggs from the ovaries is blocked. In addition, like all progestins, it thickens cervical mucus, suppresses the growth of endometrial tissue, and alters tubal motility.

Administration

It is recommended that Depo-Provera be administered in a dosage of 150 mg given intramuscularly every three months (thirteen weeks) with no added estrogen. It is important that it be delivered deeply into muscle; if it is left in subcutaneous or fatty tissue it may not be absorbed consistently. Attempts to increase the dosage and give injections every six months resulted in lower rates of effectiveness in some studies.

DMPA is given as a suspension of micronized crystals that dissolve and are gradually absorbed. Blood levels go up immediately after the injection and then gradually decline. The 150 mg dose provides protection for up to four months; women are told to get their next injection in three months, thus there is a two- to four-week grace period if they are late in getting their next shot. However, if the interval between injections is more than thirteen weeks, pregnancy must be ruled out before giving the next dose. When women discontinue the use of this agent, their blood levels of DMPA decrease gradually after the last injection, becoming undetectable after three to nine months. Clearance has been shown to be slower in heavier women.

The first injection of Depo-Provera should be given within the first five days after the onset of a normal menstrual period to avoid administration during an early unrecognized pregnancy, although there is no evidence of any damage to a fetus when this has happened inadvertently. If the first injection is given more than five days after the beginning of menses, a backup method of contraception such as male latex condoms should be used for several weeks because the next ovulation may not be inhibited. Similarly, DMPA should be given within five days after a pregnancy termination. Following a term delivery, DMPA may be started within the first five days postpartum if a woman is not breast-feeding or at six weeks if she is. Unlike the combined OCs, Depo-Provera, given immediately after delivery, does not interfere with lactation; in fact, it actually increases the flow of breast milk, stimulates an increased amount of protein in the milk, and allows for longer periods of breast-feeding. Although very small amounts of DMPA can be found in breast milk, there has never been any evidence that they pose any danger to nursing infants.

Effectiveness

Depo-Provera is one of the most effective contraceptive methods developed to date, fewer than one pregnancy per year per hundred women being reported. It is unique in that perfect and average use-effectiveness rates, both over 99 percent, are almost identical. Moreover, due to its prolonged duration of action, even those individuals who are one to two weeks late in returning for their next injection are rarely found to have become pregnant. Also, the protection against unwanted pregnancy given by the use of DMPA is not adversely affected by factors such as body weight. Finally, it is as effective as IUDs and implants and, long-term, is likely to be more effective than female sterilization.

Advantages

Depo-Provera provides safe and highly effective long-term protection. Continuation rates are, in general, better than with OCs and barriers, ranging from 50 percent to 89 percent at the end of the first year, according to a number of different studies. Women are not required to use a method of birth control with every act of sexual intercourse, a practice often disliked by both men and women. Moreover, they do not have to remember to take a pill every day; we know only too well that women forget to take their pills, take them incorrectly, and often discontinue their use without obtaining another method of birth control. It has repeatedly been shown that compliance, continuation, and average-use pregnancy rates for methods requiring repetitive behavior are always much lower than the perfect-use effectiveness rates for those same methods might suggest.

Since DMPA contains no estrogen, it has no estrogen side effects and may be used safely by women who have a history of abnormal blood clotting or thromboembolism, those over thirty-five who smoke and should not use OCs, and those with certain types of congenital heart disease. It may also be used by women who have migraine headaches, hypertension, systemic lupus erythematosus, and possibly liver disease.

The total progestin dose in Depo-Provera is much lower than that in a pill containing the same hormone, inasmuch as the injectable route avoids the peak-and-trough levels that are needed with daily oral administration, the peak levels being higher than necessary in order that the trough levels remain high enough to maintain effectiveness. DMPA has shown no adverse effects on immune responses and on vitamin and mineral metabolism. There are minimal effects on blood lipids but no clinically significant metabolic changes have been found. No adverse effects on blood vessels have been noted and there has been no increase in cardiovascular morbidity or mortality. Use of Depo-Provera has not resulted in either hypertension or thromboembolic complications.

Because, like the OCs, it decreases the amount of menstrual blood loss, DMPA not only lowers the incidence of but also produces an improvement in iron-deficiency anemia. Because it very effectively blocks ovulation, it relieves many menstrual symptoms, such as dysmenorrhea, that occur with ovulatory cycles. Interestingly, it also appears to reduce the severity of sickle-cell disease by increasing hemoglobin levels and red blood cell survival and by decreasing the frequency of the painful crises that are a major part of this disease.

Also, because of the sedative properties of progestins, DMPA is valuable for women who suffer from seizure disorders.

Depo-Provera offers other benefits such as a reduced risk of cancer of the uterus and (probably) the ovary, fewer ectopic pregnancies and ovarian cysts, fewer uterine fibroids, less vaginal candidiasis (monilia), and a probable decreased risk of PID. Women with endometriosis have been treated with DMPA for many years so, as might be expected, there is a lower incidence of this disease during Depo-Provera administration. Women taking anticonvulsant drugs that have been shown to reduce the effectiveness of low-dose OCs are also good candidates for DMPA use. Moreover, women taking prescription drugs known to have serious adverse fetal effects, such as Accutane (given for the treatment of severe acne), need to use a highly effective form of birth control such as Depo-Provera. Finally, long-term users have not been found to have any significant adverse side effects and therefore age is not a limitation. Thus, it appears that DMPA has a wide margin of safety and no deaths as yet have ever been reported that were proved to be due to its administration.

For some women, whether for personal or cultural reasons, the use of a method that is entirely private is of key importance. Unlike OCs, implants, barriers, and even IUDs, the choice of DMPA ensures almost total confidentiality. Finally, Depo-Provera is particularly useful in those areas of the world that have a severe shortage of good comprehensive health-care facilities.

Bleeding Patterns

It has been well known for many years that women taking DMPA have an increased incidence of abnormal menstrual cycles in the first six to nine months of use. Irregular menses with occasional heavy bleeding is reported by 15 to 20 percent of users. However, due to the effects of the progestin on the endometrium, in time there is a progressive increase in the number of women who develop amenorrhea (no menstrual periods) as the endometrial tissues become thinner and thinner. About half of all users cease to bleed after one year, and even more with continued use. Many women, particularly teenagers, like this side effect; some even look forward to this possibility once they are reassured that they are not pregnant and will suffer no ill effects.

It is very important to warn women in advance about the changes that they will probably have in their normal bleeding patterns. They need to be told that heavy irregular bleeding is usually temporary. If it becomes a real problem, there are several ways to treat it, once local pathology has been ruled out. Estrogen may be given for two to three weeks, OCs may be prescribed for one to two cycles, or ibuprofen taken for five to seven days. These treatments are often of help but the bleeding problems frequently return after stopping their use.

Cultural Attitudes

Women's attitudes toward bleeding and spotting (and also men's) vary considerably depending on their cultural background. Hindu women cannot prepare food and Muslim women cannot pray if they are bleeding. These two groups and also Orthodox Jews are not allowed to have intercourse if vaginal bleeding, whatever the cause, is present.

It is not surprising that vaginal bleeding is almost always viewed so negatively. Surveys of many languages, looking for words related to menses, have found them to be almost uniformly unpleasant—"the curse" or some variant thereof is nearly universal.

Many women (and even more men) regard intercourse during vaginal bleeding to be distasteful, unhygienic, uncomfortable, dangerous, or dirty. Long and/or frequent episodes of menstrual irregularities such as are common early in the use of Depo-Provera may have a profound effect on sexual relations. This often leads to discontinuation, as has been noted with all other contraceptive methods that result in abnormal bleeding patterns.

There are still some areas of the world where bleeding women are actually viewed with fear; it is believed that the food they cook will make the people who eat it get sick, that the water in lakes that they walk by will become poisonous, and that men with whom they have sexual relations will develop strange illnesses and possibly die. In some places bleeding women are still being banished to "menstrual huts." Social scientists who have studied this cultural phenomena report that these women, freed of their domestic reponsibilities, are relaxed and very happy; they rest, make beautiful tapestries, and are almost always somewhat reluctant to return home to their villages.

In the past, conventional wisdom has held—and usually still does—that women needed to bleed regularly. There are a number of cultural myths about menstrual periods. One of the most common of these is the belief of some women that they must bleed a certain number of days every month to get rid of unclean vapors and dirty blood that would otherwise build up in their bodies.

However, there is some reason to question the validity of a woman's natural need for regular menstrual periods. A recently published highly controversial book suggests that menstruation may actually be obsolete, and that amenorrhea is really highly desirable for most women. Also, new approaches to OC use are being explored in attempts to decrease the number of bleeding episodes.

Most important, it has always been found that good counseling prior to treatment and particularly in the event of the development of adverse side effects such as abnormal bleeding and amenorrhea will do much to relieve anxiety and improve compliance and continuation rates.

Disadvantages

The use of Depo-Provera carries with it minor nonserious side effects very similar to those associated with the use of OCs. They include breast tenderness, abdominal bloating, headache, depression, dizziness, nervousness, fatigue, reduced libido, and hair loss. These reported complaints are usually not severe or long-lasting and may or may not have been due to the use of DMPA. One side effect originally reported was weight gain; more than half of the women noted this during the first six months of use. The weight gain averaged four to five pounds per year for about three years after which it leveled off. On the other hand, some 20 to 40 percent of women were found to lose weight. More recent studies have failed to show weight gain as a consistent side effect; it is most often related to poor dietary habits, lack of exercise, and growing older.

As in the case of the other hormonal agents, DMPA provides no protection against the transmission of STDs and HIV/AIDS. This fact must be made clear to all DMPA users.

Cancer

International studies on Depo-Provera and the possible induction of malignancy have been conducted in many areas over the course of many years. In 1979, the WHO Collaborative Study of Neoplasia and Steroid Contraceptives was begun in Kenya, Thailand, and Mexico, and was carried out for nine years. Results from this study and a number of others showed no increased risk of ovarian, endometrial, cervical, breast, or liver cancer. In fact, in a number of programs a reduction in the risk of endometrial cancer and possibly ovarian cancer was noted. The WHO study found that DMPA use sharply lowered the risk of endometrial cancer for at least eight years following the last injection, the protection offered being even greater than that seen with OCs.

The only residual area of concern regarding the possible association of a malignancy with DMPA use, raised at the time of the 1992 FDA meeting, was related to breast cancer. Research carried out at Emory University in 1980 and the CDC in 1983 had found no increased risk, even with prolonged use. In 1989, a paper from New Zealand reported a slightly increased relative risk in women under of the age of twenty-five; however, there was no overall increase in risk over time. The previously mentioned WHO study, published in 1991, showed a very slightly increased risk in the first four years of use, but no long-term effects. In 1995, all of the data from the WHO and New Zealand studies were pooled and reevaluated; they showed no overall increased risk of breast cancer in DMPA users. A single exception was a possible slight increase seen in women who had had only one injection, which was of debatable scientific importance.

The data presented at the FDA hearing suggested three possible reasons for these findings. First, short-term use was most common in younger women under the age of thirty-five, who normally have a low incidence of breast cancer. Second, DMPA may have stimulated the growth of preexisting tumors, particularly in this age group. Third, there may have been enhanced detection of the tumors, since these women were receiving regular medical care. Most importantly, if DMPA actually caused breast cancer—the matter of greatest concern—one would have expected an increased rate with prolonged use. This, in fact, did not occur.

Osteoporosis

Aside from the continuing issue of breast cancer, only two other possibly significant concerns were raised at the FDA meeting. The first of these was the potential induction of osteoporosis. The question was stimulated by a report from New Zealand regarding decreased bone density in a small group of thirty long-term (at least five years) continuous DMPA users. The measurements obtained were found to be intermediate between those of thirty untreated women before their menopause and a group of thirty postmenopausal women with some bone loss. There was no clinical evidence of osteoporosis and no fractures occurred. Moreover, with longer periods of use, the bone loss did not increase. Also, these bone changes disappeared and the bone density measurements returned to normal after stopping the administration of Depo-Provera.

While the findings in this study were disturbing, careful review of the details of the study protocol showed some rather significant omissions. First, no pretreatment bone density analyses were done for comparative purposes; baseline information that would have permitted a more accurate assessment of the possible impact of the administration of DMPA to these women was not available. Second, the study did not analyze for such things as diet and exercise, nor were medical histories taken which included data on pregnancies and any problems relating to menstrual abnormalities, especially amenorrhea. Finally, and particularly important, it turned out that more DMPA users were smokers than the women in the other two groups. All of these factors are known to increase the risk of osteoporosis. The FDA felt that the findings of this study warranted additional investigation but that they were not, in themselves, a reason to deny approval.

The one residual concern in this regard is the observation, reported in 1995, that a study of close to fifty adolescents (twelve to twenty-one years old) showed a 1.5 percent decrease in bone density in the first year of DMPA use. Their x-ray findings were compared to those obtained from three other groups of the same age—oral contraceptive users, subdermal implant wearers, and adolescents taking no hormones. The subjects in all three of these groups showed a 3 percent increase in their bone densities. Because this is the age at which girls normally increase their bone mass, these findings were especially worthy of concern. Unfortunately, long-term data on the possible adverse effects of DMPA administration in this age group are not yet available and thus additional carefully controlled studies are being done.

This particular report has caused some health-care providers to avoid the use of DMPA in very young (twelve- to fourteen-year-old) girls until more information becomes available. Parenthetically, it has been pointed out that estrogen levels are higher in this group than those found in young girls who exercise excessively to the point where they stop having menstrual periods and begin to lose bone and develop fractures. In addition, attempts have been made to try to assess the risk/benefit ratio of DMPA use with that of having a baby; pregnancy is known to produce a much larger drain on bone minerals, another major reason to prevent unwanted pregnancies in this particular population. Fortunately the replacement of bone loss is very rapid in young girls, and the use of calcium supplements and proper diet have been shown to markedly increase bone mass in this age group.

Future Fertility

Many studies have shown that most users of Depo-Provera have a delay in the return of ovulation and fertility. At six months after stopping their injections, about 50 percent of women have begun to ovulate, at twelve months 75 percent, and at twenty-four months 82 percent. Among women attempting to become pregnant, the median time to ovulation and conception has been found to be about ten months. Two thirds conceive by the end of one year and almost 95 percent within eighteen to twenty-four months following their last injection. These rates are not related to the duration of use.

It is important to note that the ultimate return of fertility is essentially the same as that found with all other contraceptive agents and that pregnancy rates eventually are similar to those seen in women who have used no form of birth control at all. However, because of the predictable delay, women using DMPA who are planning a future pregnancy should be advised to stop their injections a year before they want to conceive.

Fetal Effects

The second concern expressed at the FDA hearings dealt with infants born as the result of accidental pregnancies that occurred within the first four weeks after an injection with DMPA. These babies were observed to have somewhat lower birth weights, but no long-term adverse effects were found when follow-up data were obtained. Moreover, the overall risk was judged to be very low because pregnancies with the correct use of Depo-Provera are exceedingly rare. Also a group of babies inadvertently exposed to Depo-Provera in utero have been carefully monitored up to the time of their adolescence; no physical, mental, or behavioral abnormalities have been found.

Contraindications

The suggested contraindications for DMPA are similar to those for OCs. They include known or suspected pregnancy, unexplained abnormal vaginal bleeding, reproductive tract and breast malignancies, severe cardiovascular disease, thromboembolic disorders, depression, and liver disease. However, only the first two of these are viewed today by most investigators to be absolute; the others fall into the category of relative contraindications with varying degrees of importance, as more data become available that will allow a better determination of the actual risks.

Usage

Discontinuation rates of Depo-Provera are very similar for adult women and adolescents. About one-third stop by the end of one year, and one-half by two years. In one study of fifty teenagers, more than two-thirds were continuing their DMPA use at one year, half at two years, and only 18 percent at three years. The reasons for discontinuations were found to differ, but they were usually related to changes in bleeding patterns. While episodes of irregular bleeding bothered both groups equally, the loss of periods disturbed many of the adults but was cited as highly desirable by 72 percent of the adolescents. Teenage discontinuations due to side effects are less common than with Norplant. Moreover, in a recently published study of 122 adolescents under the age of eighteen who had just given birth, users of Depo-Provera were found to have better continuation rates and fewer repeat pregnancies at one year than those selecting OCs.

Depo-Provera use has proved to be of particular value in a number of special situations. These include women who either do not like or have contraindications for other methods, women who have had a number of prior contraceptive failures, and women who wish to delay sterilization. It is also useful in the control of excessive menses and for women who find amenorrhea either acceptable or desirable. Moreover, it has been found to be very valuable for pregnancy prevention in the severely mentally retarded, frequent victims of sexual abuse. In the past many of these women have had hysterectomies in order to control their significant menstrual hygiene problems.

Depo-Provera is also often the method of choice for individuals with severe neuroses and psychoses, alcoholics, and substance abusers, all of whom have poor records of compliance with the use of OCs and barrier contraceptives. In the past, the prevailing wisdom was that teenagers and women who have not yet had children should not be given DMPA. However, more recent studies show that if these women want long-term highly effective protection against unwanted pregnancies—and they are properly counseled, particularly about the delay in the return of fertility—there is no reason to withhold the use of Depo-Provera.

Fortunately, DMPA has, so far, not suffered from the intense media and legal attacks launched against the OCs (and particularly

Norplant) that have proved to be so destructive. As a result, the fear of litigation has not been a significant deterrent to the use of Depo-Provera.

New Injectables

Several other progestin-only injectable regimens have been studied in recent years. DMPA, given in 250 to 300 mg doses every six months, has been used in a number of countries where it has been found to be highly effective. The WHO Task Force on Long-Acting Agents for the Regulation of Fertility has done large trials of a product called Noristerat; it contains 200 mg of norethindrone enanthate and is given every two months. These trials show that Noristerat is as effective as 150 mg DMPA given every three months. A major advantage of this progestin is the fact that regular menses are found in 60 percent of women at one year, gradually increasing to 75 percent at three years. Also, in most cases, fertility returns to pretreatment levels in six months after stopping the drug.

Two additional progestin-only injectables currently are being evaluated by WHO. They are levonorgestrel cyclobutylcarboxylate and levonorgestrel butanoate. Both offer several months of protection. In doses of 12.5 mg, ovulation is suppressed for two to three months; doses of 25 mg block ovulation for five to six months. Doses of 50 mg are effective for more than eight months.

Attempts to control bleeding problems have led to the development of new injectables that contain estrogen as well as a progestin. It has been shown that abnormal bleeding is less and continuation rates are better with their use than with DMPA alone.

Also, for a number of years, the need for monthly injectables has been expressed by a number of clinicians; several of these products have been developed and are currently in use in other countries. They are as effective as DMPA but have much better cycle control and a more rapid return of fertility. Two of these are hydroxyprogesterone caproate (250 mg) plus estradiol cypionate (5 mg), currently being used in China, and dihydroxyprogesterone acetophenide (150 mg) and estradiol enanthate (10 mg), used in Latin America.

In 1993, after conducting several clinical trials, WHO reported the use of two additional combined monthly injectables. The first is 25 mg medroxyprogesterone acetate (DMPA) and 5 mg estradiol cypionate (MPA/E2C). This contraceptive was previously called Cyclofem or Cyclo-Provera and is currently named Lunelle™. It has been studied for more than thirty years and given to 7,927 women in Thailand, Indonesia, Tunisia, Jamaica, and Mexico. It is very effective; ovulation is suppressed for about forty-two days but normal cycles continue. It is rapidly reversible and has no serious adverse side effects. The initial injection should be given within the first five days after the start of a normal menstrual period. It can also be given within the first ten days after a first-trimester pregnancy termination, and between four to six weeks postpartum. Repeat injections are given every twenty-eight to thirty days, with an outside range of twenty-three to thirty-three days.

The usual contraindications to the use of estrogen apply in this case including not administering the product to lactating women and to those over the age of thirty-five who smoke. It is quite possible that the noncontraceptive health benefits found with the use of OCs may also be observed with the administration of MPA/E2C. Its efficacy rates are as good as those of DMPA and it produces fewer bleeding problems. This product has been introduced in a number of countries where it has been well accepted. It received FDA approval in October 2000 and is now available for general use in the United States.

A similar product known as Mesigyna is also given once a month. It contains 50 mg norethisterone enanthate and 5 mg estradiol valerate and is very effective.

Both of these monthly injectables have failure rates of less than 1 percent and have lower rates of irregular and prolonged bleeding as well as fewer missed periods and lower rates of amenorrhea compared to DMPA. Even though the bleeding problems were less common, they still accounted for most of the discontinuations. Some women view injections given monthly rather than every three months as an advantage; for others this represents a disadvantage.

Another approach, one studied for a number of years, uses one or more hormones incorporated in microcapsules, microspheres, or pellets. Some of these are biodegradable, which means they do not have to be surgically removed. One of these pellets, about the size of a grain of rice, contains 90 percent norethindrone and 10 percent cholesterol. The pellets release a contraceptive level of the progestin for twelve to eighteen months and then begin to disintegrate; they are completely used up after two years. In addition, studies have been carried out on two, three, and four different pellets, the last group having the highest incidence of amenorrhea and rate of suppression of ovulation. The pellets can be removed for a few months after insertion but not thereafter because of disintegration. As in the case of all other hormonal methods, bleeding problems (irregular bleeding and/or amenorrhea) are the main reason for discontinuation. Unlike Depo-Provera, ovulation and fertility return quite promptly, in most cases within two to three months after the last injection.

One of the microspheres being studied is made of a polymer that is also used for biodegradable sutures. The microspheres range in size from 0.06 to 0.1 mm in diameter and currently use preparations containing 65 or 100 mg of norethindrone. They produce blood levels comparable to those found with low-dose OCs. However, because of the sustained release rather than the intermittent oral doses, the hormone levels are more constant. Some of the products under study contain ethinyl estradiol in addition to the progestin. The microspheres are preloaded in a syringe in a suspension of dextran and must be thoroughly mixed prior to use. Intramuscular injection offers a sustained release of the hormone(s) over periods of one, three, or six months, depending on the formulation. The dosage and duration of action are controlled by the size and number of the spheres and the amount of hormone(s) that they contain.

The microspheres have certain advantages over the Norplant System. They are easy to inject and do not involve a surgical procedure. Also, stopping means only that no further injections are given, whereas Norplant discontinuations involve surgery and can, if the insertion was not properly done, be difficult. On the other hand, once the microspheres are injected, they cannot be removed if significant side effects or an accidental pregnancy occur. The FDA once considered the inability to remove biodegradable products a potential problem, but this issue has now been pretty much resolved.

5

Intrauterine Devices

History

IT IS BELIEVED that the first users of intrauterine devices (IUDs) were female camels. Somehow, ancient Turk and Arab caravan drivers learned that putting pebbles into the uteri of their pack animals before their long treks across the Sahara would prevent the animals from mating. Once the pebbles were removed, the female camels were once again willing to accept the sexual advances of the males. This observation was reported in French medical literature many years ago. Despite this, considerable time was to elapse before the same approach to reversible contraception was attempted in the human female.

The use of IUDs was noted by Hippocrates, and the Islamic scientist Avicenna reported the use of contraceptive pessaries as early as the eleventh century. Over the years, pessaries were fashioned from wood, glass, metals, pewter, ebony, and even diamond-studded platinum. They reportedly were used not only for contraception, but also to hold up prolapsed uteri and to induce abortions.

Development

In the more modern era, for the past 150 years, women have used numerous types of devices inserted into their uteri to prevent unwanted pregnancies. The first attempts were made in the 1800s, which resulted in the development of stem pessaries. These were small button-shaped devices that blocked the opening of the cervix and had a portion—the stem—that went up through the cervical canal into the uterine cavity. In 1902, Hollweg in Germany manufactured one of these devices. It was to be inserted by the woman herself for protection against unwanted pregnancy. However, it caused a number of infections and was soon discarded.

In the early part of the twentieth century, a different approach was developed. Rings made of silkworm, catgut, silver, gold, and steel were introduced in Germany by Richard Richter and Ernest Gräfenberg. One of Richter's devices, described in 1909, had a nickel and bronze wire that was brought out through the cervix into the vagina, reportedly causing damage to sexual partners. K. Pust then combined this type of ring with a pessary and changed to a catgut tail. This device was widely used in Germany during World War I.

Some years later, Gräfenberg stopped using IUD tails because he believed that they caused infections. His tailless IUDs enjoyed a brief period of popularity until the Nazis, who were opposed to birth control, came into power. Gräfenberg, who was Jewish, was sent to jail but managed to escape to New York City, where he died in 1955. At about the same time as Gräfenberg was developing his IUDs, gold- and silver-plated rings were designed by Ota in Japan. He retained the ring configuration but added a hub and spokes in the center, believing that this would reduce the expulsion rate, which was quite high with the Gräfenberg rings. He also thought that this design would reduce the chance of bowel obstruction if perforation of the device into the abdomen were to occur, allowing a loop of intestine to be caught in the hole in the center of the ring. He, too, ran into political problems during World War II and was exiled.

The popularity of the IUD waxed and waned. The initial enthusiasm they generated, particularly in Europe, gradually disappeared when major concerns again arose about a possible association with pelvic infections. This concern was heightened by a worldwide pandemic of gonorrhea in the 1930s, part of the blame for which was ascribed to IUD use.

Interest picked up again, however, in 1959, stimulated by favorable reports from Oppenheimer in Israel and Ishihama in Japan. Shortly afterward, because of increasing concerns about the rapid growth of population and the equally rapid dwindling of natural resources, the Population Council, established by John D. Rockefeller III at the Rockefeller University in New York City, invited them to present their studies. Their results were so impressive that programs were soon started in the United States to develop, study, and begin to use the next generation of IUDs.

Current IUDs

The earliest intrauterine devices developed in the modern era were made of a plastic, polyethylene, in a variety of different shapes. A major technological advance—the ability to give memory to plastic— made these new IUDs possible: they were molded in the desired final form; their shape was altered during the insertion process, but the original configuration was restored once the IUD was in the uterine cavity. Another innovation, begun at that time, was the addition of barium to the plastic so that the IUD would show up in an x-ray. The first such device, the Margulies Coil, was introduced in 1960. Shortly thereafter, several other plastic IUDs were invented, including the Birnberg bow, the Lem, and the Dalkon Shield. The Lippes Loops were made by Ortho Pharmaceuticals from 1964 to 1985 in four sizes; at about the same time the Saf-T-Coil was made in two sizes.

In 1962, the Population Council held the first international conference on IUDs. Dr. Jack Lippes presented the data on his devices, and the Lippes Loops began to be widely used all over the world. Shortly after the IUD conference, the Cooperative Statistical Program (CSP) was set up by the Population Council under the leadership of Dr. Christopher Tietze. Data were gathered on 27,000 insertions of IUDs of various types. Detailed statistical analyses were carried out looking at pregnancy, perforation and expulsion rates, the reasons for removal, and possible side effects.

Several years of study by the CSP and the Pathfinder Fund revealed that although these newer IUDs were quite effective, they had higher than anticipated rates of perforation and expulsion. Even more importantly, they caused significant cramping and bleeding, which often led to removal. Several investigators believed that these problems were directly related to the large size of the devices. They put pressure on the walls of the uterus (which caused the uterus to cramp in an attempt to expel the foreign body) and on the endometrium (producing erosion and bleeding). Parenthetically, the Margulies Coil had its own special side effect; it had a hard plastic tail which protruded through the cervix, which could cause considerable discomfort to male partners if the tail was left too long at the time of insertion.

Another new approach involved stainless steel springs, which were compressed for insertion and subsequently reopened in the uterus. Two examples were the Majzlin Spring and the "M" (M-shaped) device. While these devices proved very effective at preventing pregnancy, they often embedded deeply into the uterine wall and were extremely difficult to remove. As a result, their distribution was limited and brief.

Concerns about the large size of the earlier plastic devices led to the development of the smaller T-shaped IUDs. Dr. Howard Tatum, the originator of the copper-Ts at the Population Council, believed that a "T" platform would fit the shape of the uterine cavity whereas the larger devices forced the uterus to conform to them, which caused side effects. Although these new T-shaped IUDs produced fewer bleeding and cramping problems, Tatum found that when used alone, they had unacceptably high failure rates. During further research efforts, however, he met Jaime Zipper, who was working in Chile, studying the use of various metals for contraception. Many different metals were studied and finally copper was selected for a number of reasons, one of which was its local effects on the endometrium. In a collaborative effort, they showed that the addition of copper wire to the T platform would reduce the pregnancy rates to very acceptable levels.

As studies continued, the amount of copper was progressively increased and the pregnancy rates improved proportionately. The first of these devices, the TCu-200 (200 mm^2 of exposed copper wire wound around the stem), was developed by Tatum and sold by Finishing Enterprises. A similar device known as the Tatum-T™ was sold by G. D. Searle and Company. Another IUD, the Cu-7, which was shaped like a "7," also had copper wire wound around its stem. It was developed in 1971 and rapidly achieved wide popularity. These and virtually all of the subsequently developed IUDs had monofilament tails that were brought out through the cervix into the vagina.

The only FDA-approved copper IUD currently available in the United States is the TCu-380A (the A indicates the addition of copper to the two arms) known as the ParaGard™, sold first by GynoPharma and now by Ortho-McNeil Pharmaceutical, Inc. It has a flexible T-shaped frame made of polyethylene with copper wire wound around the vertical stem; an additional amount of copper is provided by two sleeves, one around each of the two horizontal arms of the device, giving a total amount of 380 mm² of copper. It received FDA approval in November 1984.

The ParaGard™ proved to be the most effective IUD ever developed, with a failure rate in the first year of use of less than 1 percent. This made it comparable to Depo-Provera, Norplant, and male and female sterilization; better than OCs; and far better than the barrier methods. The FDA originally approved the use of the ParaGard™ for four years, extending this to six in 1989 and to eight in 1991; it is currently approved for ten years and may go to twelve years of use. Thus, it has the longest duration of contraceptive action of any of the currently available long-term reversible methods of family planning.

A number of other copper-bearing IUDs have been and continue to be manufactured around the world. They include the Gyne T™ (Canada), TCu 220C (Canada, Finland), TCu 380 Ag (Finland), Nova T™ (Finland, Sweden), Multiload (Switzerland), and Sterlys™ (France). They are mainly T-shaped in design, contain 200 to 380 mm² of copper, and have estimated durations of action ranging from three to twenty years. Another type of IUD was developed in the late 1960s and was introduced in 1976—the Progesterone-T intrauterine device—marketed by the Alza Corporation as the Progestasert ™. It also has a T-shaped plastic platform, which measures 36 × 32 mm, but in this case there is a reservoir of 38 mg of progesterone mixed with barium in the vertical stem. A monofilament nylon thread is attached to the bottom of the stem to aid in identification and removal. Each device releases 65 mg of progesterone per day—the total progesterone is enough to provide protection for one year. It reduces menstrual blood loss because of the action of the progesterone on the endometrium, which makes it particularly valuable for women who experience excessive menses. However, it has a failure rate of almost 3 percent, has a slightly higher rate of ectopic pregnancy, and has the added disadvantage that it has be replaced annually. As a result, it has never been widely used and will soon be taken off the market.

Dalkon Shield

Just when intrauterine contraception was becoming increasingly well accepted in the 1960s and early 1970s, it suffered a serious setback as the result of the disastrous effects of the Dalkon Shield episode. This IUD was made in the form of a shield with multiple small projecting side arms, which helped to anchor it in the uterine cavity. It was introduced in the United States in 1970 by A. H. Robins. The first indication of trouble was the publication of an article by Dr. Donald Christian in 1974, documenting several maternal deaths due to septic (infected) mid-trimester spontaneous abortions, some with the use of Dalkon Shields. As a result, a number of studies were undertaken, looking into the possibility of these infections being IUD-related.

Ultimately, the studies determined that the Dalkon Shield posed a disproportionately higher risk than all of the other IUDs. Tatum determined the cause for this in detailed laboratory studies. He found that the multifilament tail of the Shield had a wicking action, which allowed bacteria from the vagina to be carried up into the uterus; all of the other marketed IUDs had a single (monofilament) tail.

Previously conducted research had shown that the mucus in the endocervical canal had antibacterial action. This protected against ascending infections when a monofilament tail was used but clearly had no impact on a tail containing hundreds of filaments enclosed in a plastic sheath, as was the case with the Shield. The results of this research plus the growing clinical evidence about the dangers posed by the use of the Dalkon Shield led to an FDA review and its removal from the market in the United States in 1975. In the early 1980s, the FDA recommended that all Dalkon Shield devices then in use be removed. Although the manufacturer could potentially have replaced the multifilament tail with one made of monofilament, this was never done, possibly because a heavy tail was needed for removal because of the embedding of the multiple sidearms. Most unfortunately, the impact of this disaster on intrauterine contraception was and continues to be immense in the United States.

Mechanisms of Action

Over the years, there have been many theories as to the mechanisms of action of intrauterine devices. One of the earliest theories was that they led to the development of an inflammatory response of the type common to all foreign bodies, producing an infection which prevented implantation of a fertilized egg. A second theory, based on studies in the monkey, was that IUDs increased the activity of the Fallopian tubes, propelling eggs into the uterus before they could be fertilized. Finally, it was thought, but never documented, that the devices somehow upset the user's normal hormonal balance.

A more recent school of thought, predominant for a number of years, was that the local changes which were found in the endometrial cavities of IUD users accounted for the effectiveness of these devices. Many biochemical changes in the endometrial fluids as well as the appearance of numerous white blood cells were documented. These alterations were believed to act in one or more of three ways, first to damage a fertilized egg, second to prevent implantation, or third, to disrupt an early pregnancy.

It is particularly important, given our current heated and confrontational political environment, to recognize that we now know that the mechanisms of action of IUDs are quite different from what we have believed in the past, i.e., that they acted as abortifacients. Newer data from many studies indicate that this is not the case; they show that IUDs actually have contraceptive action prior to fertilization, which must take place in the upper portion of the fallopian tube, and therefore do not act by interrupting established pregnancies.

Specific biochemical and enzymatic changes in the uterine tissues and fluids have been found with all IUDs—nonmedicated plastic as well as copper—and hormone-bearing devices. They all set up a sterile foreign-body inflammatory response which is spermicidal; this is the primary mechanism of action of the plastic devices. Copper-bearing IUDs produce the same types of endometrial responses as the non-medicated devices; however, the reactions are much more intense. Copper also has a direct toxic effect on sperm, in the cervical mucus, the uterine cavity, and the fallopian tubes. In fact, all of the findings noted here probably act together to make copper IUDs an extremely effective form of contraception.

The progesterone-bearing devices have been found to have basically the same effects in the uterus. In addition, the release of their hormonal content produces a direct action on the endometrium and also thickens the mucus in the cervix, blocking the passage of some of the sperm. Those that succeed in getting into the uterus are acted on by the progesterone, which destroys their ability to fertilize an egg. In addition, the hormone, when it is absorbed in small amounts, may partially suppress the development of eggs in the ovaries, which helps to prevent ovulation.

There is a large body of additional new scientific evidence documenting the fact that IUDs act primarily as contraceptives. For example, laboratory tests have detected no pregnancy hormone, human chorionic gonadotropin (hCG), in the blood of women wearing IUDs. A fertilized egg begins to produce this hormone around the time of implantation. Very sensitive hormone assays have failed to find it in almost all IUD wearers.

Studies of the contents of fallopian tubes revealed important changes. In women who were wearing IUDs, no normally developing fertilized eggs were present in their fallopian tubes when they were exposed to pregnancy at the time of ovulation, whereas fertilized eggs were found in almost half of the samples taken from women using no form of contraception. In addition, almost no viable sperm were found in the tubes of women with IUDs in place.

Fewer unfertilized eggs were obtained from the tubes of IUD wearers compared to nonwearers, the decrease being most marked when copper devices were used. Furthermore, when uterine and tubal fluids from these women were examined, many white blood cells and small amounts of copper were found in both fluids, showing that materials in the uterine cavity can migrate up into the tubes. It is well known that fertilization is severely adversely affected by changes in the chemical composition of both of these fluids. Finally, it has also been documented that IUD users have fewer ectopic pregnancies than nonusers. In fact, one study showed a 60 percent reduction in the incidence of ectopic pregnancies in IUD wearers. All of these observations further support the evidence for certain mechanisms of action that occur outside the uterine cavity, exerting contraceptive effects before fertilization can occur in the tubes.

Effectiveness

IUDs are one of the most effective forms of reversible contraception available today. Copper IUDs have a failure rate of less than 1 percent, which is comparable to and actually better than the long-term results found in recent studies of tubal ligation. The Progestasert™ has a failure rate of about 3 percent.

The overall effectiveness of any method of birth control is, in the larger sense, also a matter of patient acceptance and continuation of use. In this regard also, IUDs are very effective; continuation rates at one year are far better than with barriers and oral contraceptives, and with each year of use, the rates continue to increase. To some degree, this may be due to the fact that it is easy to discontinue taking OCs or using barriers, whereas stopping contraception with an IUD requires a conscious decision and the intervention of a health-care provider.

Insertion

Techniques

Not only have IUDs themselves undergone considerable improvements in recent years, but the techniques of their insertion have improved as well. The older nonmedicated plastic devices were inserted using a "push-out" technique. The IUD was stretched out, introduced into the uterus, and then pushed upward to the top of the cavity. Then, the device returned to the original preinsertion shape. However, if these IUDs were stretched out and put into their inserters too early, they lost their memory. If they were left too low in the uterine cavity, expulsion, pregnancy, and cramping and bleeding rates were increased. A number of studies found that it was essential to have the IUD at the very top of the uterus to get the maximum protection against pregnancy and to avoid adverse side effects.

The T-shaped medicated devices currently on the market utilize a far more effective method of insertion—the withdrawal technique. The IUDs are released from their inserters only after their correct placement at the top of the uterine cavity has been determined, following which the inserter is withdrawn.

Timing

IUD insertions may be performed at any time during the menstrual cycle. For many years, it was believed that the insertion should only be done at the time of the menses. This would remove the chance of inserting an IUD into an early unrecognized pregnancy. It would also allow the bleeding due to the insertion to be discharged with the menstrual flow, thus avoiding an additional episode of bleeding at the time of an insertion carried out somewhat later. Another commonly held belief was that the opening in the cervix is widest at the time of menses; more recent studies show that maximum dilatation actually occurs around the time of ovulation.

There are several other good reasons for doing insertions at the time of ovulation. There is usually little or no bleeding and, inasmuch as blood supports the growth of bacteria, avoiding the additional blood resulting from a menstrual period may possibly decrease the risk of infection. It has also been found that midcycle insertions have been associated with fewer expulsions, less pain and bleeding, and fewer pregnancies.

An additional and very compelling reason has been found for inserting IUDs at times other than during the menstrual flow. Many nonmenstruating women asking for an IUD have been told (and agreed) to return with their next menstrual period for their insertion, but have failed to come back. If an individual is asking for an IUD, she is obviously motivated to prevent an unwanted pregnancy. Despite this fact, experience has shown that women often become distracted by other events in their lives and get pregnant before returning. In addition, a woman can be saved the inconvenience and cost of a repeat visit by an insertion performed at the time of her original request, if she is not pregnant. This can be determined with a high degree of confidence by taking her medical history, doing a pelvic examination, and then using one of the currently available highly sensitive urine pregnancy tests.

Insertion Procedure

Certain steps need to be carried out at the time of the insertion. A careful pelvic examination must be done to rule out infection and any significant anatomical abnormalities. Also, it is very important that the position of the uterus be accurately determined. Most uteri are in a fairly straight line with the cervix. However, a uterus can be sharply flexed forward (anteflexion) or backward (retroflexion).

First, the cervix is exposed with the use of a vaginal speculum. Next, the vagina and cervix are carefully cleansed with an antiseptic— either an iodine preparation or benzalkonium. Then the cervix is grasped with a specifically designed instrument and gentle traction is applied to straighten out the endocervical canal into the uterine cavity. This step is particularly important if the uterus is either markedly anteflexed or retroflexed. At this time, the distance to the top of the uterine cavity is measured using an instrument called a uterine sound, a long thin probe on which a scale is inscribed in either inches or centimeters. A uterus may be too small (less than 6 cm in depth) or too large (more than 9 cm) for the use of an IUD.

If a medicated T-shaped device is used, the IUD is inserted until it touches the top of the fundus; the IUD is then released and the inserter is removed. The tail of the device is trimmed so that it protrudes approximately two inches beyond the cervix into the vagina where it can be identified by both the user and her health-care provider. (Ultimately it will be used for the removal of the IUD.) Then the speculum is taken out of the vagina.

The insertion procedure is usually quite easy and takes about five to ten minutes. However, if the endocervical canal is found to be very tight, a local anesthetic is often injected in order to prevent pain and the possibility of fainting, which may occur as the cervix is being dilated. Many women experience mild cramping during the procedure and for a few hours thereafter and slight to moderate vaginal bleeding for the first few days after the insertion.

Removal

The reasons for removal of an IUD can be either personal or medical. A woman may make a personal choice to switch to a different contraceptive method or to stop using contraception because she wants to become pregnant or because the need for protection against pregnancy is no longer an issue. Medical indications for removal include accidental pregnancy, pelvic inflammatory disease, cramping and/or bleeding, pain on intercourse, partial expulsion, perforation, the development of uterine or cervical cancer, or the onset of menopause. In addition, it may be necessary to remove an IUD because ten years have elapsed in the case of the ParaGard™ or one year for the Progestasert™. At this time, if the woman so desires, a new device can be put in immediately.

In most instances, removal is easy. A health practitioner inserts a speculum into the woman's vagina, locates the cervix and the tail of the IUD, and then applies gentle traction to the tail. If the device is known to be still present but the tail cannot be found, the health practitioner may attempt to bring the tail out through the opening of the cervix. If this is unsuccessful, a small uterine sound can be inserted into the uterine cavity to locate the device, which is then removed with a forceps or a specially designed IUD-removal instrument. Occasionally an IUD may have become deeply embedded in the uterine wall and removal may be more difficult, sometimes requiring direct visualization using sonography, or if this fails, hysteroscopy. Only rarely will surgical intervention be required.

Once an IUD is removed, fertility returns promptly, since there have been no changes in hormone levels and ovulation has continued. This is in contrast to women who stop using OCs and typically experience a short delay, and those taking Depo-Provera who usually have a fairly long delay. Most women have relatively little difficulty in becoming pregnant; about 80 percent do so within one year. This is the same rate as that of women who have used OCs and barrier methods, as well as that found in women who have used no form of contraception. Studies have shown no increase in pregnancy complications (such as spontaneous abortion, premature onset of labor, or problems at the time of delivery) following the use of an IUD and no adverse effects on their babies have been reported.

Side Effects/Complications

Cramping and Bleeding

Cramping and bleeding have been described with the use of all IUDs, more often with the older, larger devices. These symptoms account for 5 to 15 percent of requests for removal. Pain, which is temporary, is often experienced at the time of the insertion and, along with mild cramping and variable amounts of vaginal bleeding, may last up to twenty-four hours. The bleeding may not be noticed if the insertion is done during the menstrual period but will be obvious at any other time. Persistent pain, cramping, and bleeding after the first few days, however, may be an indication of infection or partial expulsion, and women with these symptoms should get prompt medical attention.

Excessive bleeding with menstrual periods and spotting and/or bleeding between periods have been noted with all intrauterine devices. For a time, particularly right after the insertion, menses may begin a day or two earlier and may last a day or two longer than usual. Excessive bleeding is most common at the time of the first menstrual period and may persist with each menses for several months. The various types of IUDs have been found to result in different amounts of bleeding. Whereas normal menstrual blood loss averages about 30–40 ml, bleeding with copper devices averages 40–50 ml and with the nonmedicated plastic devices, 60–75 ml is common. On the other hand, because of their direct hormonal effect on the endometrium, there is a decrease in the menstrual flow with the progesterone-bearing IUDs, which average 20–30 ml per cycle. These devices also have slightly higher rates of intermenstrual bleeding and spotting but, overall, there is a decrease in total blood loss, which is an advantage for women who typically have an abnormally heavy menstrual flow. In fact, for them, this may be a good reason to select this type of IUD.

Sometimes excessive bleeding will occur after several years of use, particularly of the nonmedicated IUDs. This is usually due to the deposition of material including calcium on the surface of the device, causing it to be rough and irritating. If so, the problem is easily resolved by removing it and replacing it with a new IUD, preferably a copper device.

Women have highly variable reactions to the unusual or excessive bleeding caused by IUDs. To some, it is merely an annoyance. To others, particularly in those cultures in which sexual intercourse and participation in religious ceremonies are forbidden to bleeding women, it is a matter of great concern, and often leads to requests for removal.

Expulsion

Expulsion has always been a problem with IUDs, as uterine contractions are stimulated by the presence of a foreign body. The most common time for this to occur is with the first postinsertion menses. The expulsion rates vary with the type of device; the rates are higher with the larger devices. The ParaGard™ rate ranges from 3.3 to 7.1 percent, and the Progestasert™ between 1.2 to 4.2 percent. In general, expulsion rates are higher in younger women who have not had children.

There are two types of expulsion. The first, also known as dislodgement, is partial, which means that the IUD is displaced into the lower part of the uterine cavity or into the endocervical canal. The second is complete; in this case, the entire IUD is forced out into the vagina. The signs and symptoms of partial expulsion are often excessive spotting and bleeding, sometimes accompanied by mild cramping. On pelvic examination, the strings may be found to be longer than at the time of insertion. The lower portion of the stem of the IUD may have become visible or may be felt at the opening of the cervix. Rarely, the stem of the IUD is forced through the wall of the cervix by the contractions of the uterus and the tip can be seen protruding through into the vagina.

The diagnosis of partial expulsion is usually made by pelvic exam or, sometimes, by ultrasound. The recommended management is to remove the device, then either reinsert it higher in the fundal cavity in the proper position or replace it with a new IUD. In the case of a cervical perforation, the device should be pushed up into the cervical canal and then removed. At that point a new device can be inserted if so desired. Frequently, if the device is too low in the uterine cavity to be effective, a pregnancy is the presenting sign.

Complete expulsion may be either noticed or unnoticed. It may be preceded or accompanied by uterine cramping and/or vaginal bleeding. Some women are aware of losing the device. However, others may not be, and an unnoticed expulsion is often first diagnosed by the presence of a pregnancy. In fact, about one-third of IUD-associated pregnancies follow unnoticed expulsion.

Perforation

Perforations of the IUD through the wall of the uterus have been reported with all types of IUDs, occurring in 1 to 3 percent of insertions. In many studies, a clear relationship has been established between the incidence of this complication and the skill and experience of the person performing the procedure. The most common time of perforation is at the moment of insertion, the device being pushed totally out through the uterine wall into the pelvic or abdominal cavity. This is particularly apt to occur when the uterus is bent sharply backward, the IUD being forced out through the front wall if the retroflexed position of the uterus is not recognized. Very often the person doing the insertion will realize what has happened since the inserter will have gone beyond the previously measured distance, and will therefore remove the device and place it in the proper position. Sometimes, the woman will feel a sharp pain as the perforation occurs, so that it is recognized immediately. At other times the perforation goes unnoticed until a pregnancy is diagnosed.

Far less commonly, a partial perforation is made at the time of the insertion. The IUD is then gradually forced through the wall of the uterus out into the pelvic or abdominal cavity by contractions of the uterus.

Copper devices that have perforated into the abdomen should be removed, preferably by laparoscopy, as soon as the diagnosis is made, because the copper will immediately begin to set up intense local reactions. This can cause considerable damage to the local structures such as bowel, bladder, and rectum, sometimes resulting in massive adhesions. If too much time passes, laparoscopy may become impossible because of the adhesions, leading to the need for abdominal surgery to remove the device.

It is usually recommended that noncopper IUDs also be removed, although less urgently, because they have been known to lead to infection and abscess. When a closed device such as a ring is loose in the abdominal cavity, a loop of bowel can get caught in it causing intestinal obstruction.

Lost IUD Tail

On occasion, a woman will report not being able to feel the tail of her IUD and it will be impossible to find it at the time of pelvic examination. It is essential to see if the IUD has been expelled, to locate its position if it is found to be still present, and to exclude both intrauterine and ectopic pregnancy. If a pregnancy test is negative, the woman has not noted an expulsion, and the IUD is assumed to be in place, there are several steps to find the tail of the device. First, the cervix can be probed and if the tail is located, it can often be brought back down into the vagina. If the tail is not found, ultrasound can be used to try to determine the exact location of the IUD. If the situation is still unclear, x-rays of the pelvis and lower abdomen may be taken.

If the tail is not found but the IUD is still in the uterus, a discussion should be held with the woman to see if she wants to continue the use of her device. She must be followed very carefully and instructed to watch for expulsion of the device, particularly at the time of her menstrual periods. If the studies have failed to locate the IUD, it must be assumed that it has been expelled without being noticed. If the woman wishes, another IUD can be inserted; also she can be told that the chance of expulsion is generally lower with the second device. However, the absence of the original device must be confirmed, some women reportedly having had a second device inserted based on the false assumption that the first one had been expelled.

Pregnancy

Pregnancy should be suspected if a woman has a very scanty period, misses a period, or has signs and symptoms of pregnancy. Pregnancies can occur in either the uterus or a fallopian tube. An intrauterine pregnancy in the presence of an IUD is best handled by the removal of the device as soon as the diagnosis is made. This should be done for two important reasons. First, it has been found that sometimes a device is not removed right away because the woman says that she plans to terminate the pregnancy and asks that the IUD be removed at that time. However, if she changes her mind and delays seeking follow-up care, the IUD may be irretrievable by the time of her next visit because the tail will have been drawn up into the enlarging uterus.

A second very important reason for immediately removing the IUD is that leaving it in place can have serious health consequences, including spontaneous miscarriage, rupture of the membranes, premature delivery, and stillbirth. Of greatest concern is the fact that there is a tenfold greater risk of having a second trimester spontaneous abortion if the IUD is not removed. In the case of the Dalkon Shield, the risk was even greater when the multifilament tail, full of bacteria from the vagina, was pulled up into the uterus; a number of these abortions were associated with severe infections and proved to be fatal. Thus, if a woman is wearing a device that cannot be readily removed because the tail has disappeared, she must be warned about the dangers of leaving it in—particularly the danger of serious infection—and followed very closely if she elects to continue her pregnancy.

Ectopic pregnancies can also occur with an IUD in place and are actually more common than those found to be in the uterus, since the IUD offers better protection against uterine pregnancies. Very rarely, a fertilized egg will implant on an ovary or elsewhere in the abdomen or pelvis and begin to grow, since IUDs offer virtually no protection against these types of pregnancies. In general, when abdominal pregnancies occur, they usually do not survive but a few that went unrecognized have actually gone to term—something of a medical curiosity and often a diagnostic dilemma!

An overall 50 percent reduction in total ectopic pregnancies has been reported in IUD users in various surveys. Copper IUDs provide the greatest protection against ectopic pregnancy. Their effectiveness is in direct proportion to the total amount of exposed copper surface. Progesterone-bearing IUDs have a slightly higher rate, possibly due to the effects of the hormone on the passage of a fertilized egg through the tube; slowing it may allow the pregnancy to implant in the wall of the tube.

It is critically important to investigate the possibility of an ectopic pregnancy immediately. This is a life-threatening condition, often a virtual death sentence in the absence of good medical care. If rupture of a tubal pregnancy occurs, a woman may experience lower abdominal pain, spotting, or bleeding. If a major hemorrhage results, she may go into shock. Without a prompt diagnosis and the institution of appropriate treatment, the outcome is often fatal.

No relationship has ever been found between the duration of IUD use and the risk of ectopic pregnancy, nor do IUD users have higher rates of this condition after removal of their devices.

Fetal Damage

There has never been any evidence of damage to a baby from the presence of either a plastic or copper-bearing device when the IUD has been in the uterus throughout a pregnancy, despite several fascinating anecdotal reports to the contrary—one particularly delightful story featured a baby who was born clutching an IUD in its hand and laughing!

Examinations of the placentas at the time of delivery have shown that the presence of an IUD poses no danger since it always remains extraovular (away from the baby).

Pelvic Inflammatory Disease

The biggest concern with intrauterine contraception has always been (and continues to be) that IUDs may have the potential to cause infection. The risks of this complication were greatly overestimated in the 1970s and early 1980s. Reanalyses of the earlier data showed that there was considerable bias in the risk estimates associated with IUD use. For example, comparison groups often consisted of OC and barrier users, both methods that are now known to lower the incidence of pelvic infections. Also, many physicians tended to overdiagnose PID if a woman with pelvic symptoms was found to be wearing an IUD. The risks particularly appeared to be quite high when data from the Dalkon Shield were included in the overall risk assessments. However, when the IUDs were split into categories, the infection rates for all other IUDs were found to be considerably lower.

The major reason for the development of pelvic infections with IUDs is not the device per se but the number of sexual partners a woman has while wearing her IUD, each additional one increasing the chances of STD transmission. Moreover, her risks are higher if her partner or partners also have several partners. This is of course due to the rapidly growing incidence of sexually transmitted diseases, many of them today reaching epidemic and pandemic proportions.

There is now good evidence that only in the first twenty days following insertion is there any significant increase in the risk of PID. At all other times the potential is very low to absent provided that the woman is a good candidate for IUD use. Long-term users and even women with insulin-dependent diabetes have not been found to have higher infection rates, as long as they are not exposed to STDs.

No method has ever been devised to avoid contamination of the uterine cavity at the time of insertion. However, within days the uterus is able to destroy these invaders, and any infection occurring after that time is almost always due to an acquired STD. In a recent study, no increased risk of PID was ever found in copper-bearing IUD users who were in a mutually monogamous relationship with an uninfected partner. Moreover, it has recently been noted that copper inhibits the growth of chlamydial cultures in the laboratory and that women wearing copper-bearing devices have lower levels of antibodies against chlamydia.

Efforts have been made to determine whether or not the use of prophylactic antibiotics at the time of insertion would decrease the risk of infection. One early study suggested that doing this would help to prevent PID, but subsequent surveys have shown no advantage to this practice, and at the present time there is no reason to recommend it. Indeed, the unindicated use of antibiotics always poses its own risk of drug sensitivities and bacterial resistance.

Still today, the PID argument continues. It is probably correct to conclude that the risk of infection related to IUD use is considerably lower than was originally thought and that it is limited to the first twenty days after insertion. Finally, all the current evidence points to the fact that pelvic infections are not found in women using copper devices who are at low risk for STDs.

Malignancy

Questions have been raised in the past about the possible induction of cancer of the uterus or cervix by the use of IUDs. However, multiple studies have shown that there is no difference in the rates of these diseases in women using IUDs compared with those of non-IUD wearers. Of great interest are several recent publications reporting on a reduced risk of both endometrial and invasive cervical malignancies in current or previous IUD users. Additional studies are needed to see if this is indeed true and, if so, how it can be explained.

Advantages

Modern IUDs actually come quite close to meeting the previously noted definition of the "ideal" contraceptive. They have a number of advantages for properly selected women. Primary among these is their reliability; the copper IUDs are probably the most effective form of long-term reversible contraception available today. They are also very safe; their side effects in the vast majority of instances are annoying but not life-threatening.

Contrary to most other forms of birth control, they require only a single act of motivation, at the time of requesting an insertion. Following this, there is little need for frequent medical care. The copper IUDs can remain in place for up to ten or more years. They avoid the need for constant attention such as daily pill taking and their use is unrelated to the time of sexual intercourse, which also increases their acceptability.

Use of an IUD does not interfere with physical exercise, sexual activity, or the use of tampons. The IUD's presence is usually not obvious to either the woman or her partner. The costs of IUDs are initially relatively high, but over the long term they are the most cost-effective method of contraception currently available. Insertions are generally easy and are followed by few or no significant complications. Removals are also usually quick and painless, and there is an immediate return of fertility.

Disadvantages

The major disadvantages to IUD use are the side effects that have already been described. How these are viewed can vary widely, depending on the attitudes and needs of individual women and the differences in their cultural environments.

To obtain an IUD, a woman must go to a health-care facility for insertion, a situation that may be difficult or unpleasant for some women. An additional disadvantage is the fact that not all insurance and indemnity plans cover the costs of IUDs, their insertions, follow-up care, and removals.

The most significant problem, perhaps not actually a true disadvantage, is the general perception in the United States today that IUDs are unsafe and are therefore not a viable contraceptive option.

Good Candidates for IUD Use

There are several things to consider when a woman elects to use an IUD. First, she must have anatomically normal genitalia; certain uterine abnormalities, for example, would be contraindications. Second, it is important that she be in a mutually monogamous uninfected relationship, thus having no risk of acquiring an STD. Finally, while IUD expulsions are less frequent in women who have borne children, not having had a baby does not completely rule out their use.

IUDs are an excellent choice for many smokers over the age of thirty-five, who cannot take OCs. This is also true for women with contraindications to or failure with other forms of family planning and those who have difficulty in complying with birth control methods that require close adherence to a schedule. IUDs are also an excellent temporary or permanent substitute for surgical sterilization when women and/or their partner(s) have not yet decided to opt for a permanent form of contraception, yet who want long-term reliable protection against unplanned pregnancy.

In recent years questions have been raised as to the appropriateness of some of the earlier contraindications to IUD use, such as a history of PID, ectopic pregnancy, or diabetes. Some of these are still listed in the device labeling and patient package inserts. Many investigators now believe that some of these were based much more often on unfounded fears and medicolegal concerns than on actual medical information. For example, one recent study comparing results from insulin-dependent diabetics and nondiabetic controls, both wearing copper IUDs, found no differences in pregnancy, PID, or continuation rates; therefore, it is now believed that women with either Type 1 or Type 2 diabetes may safely use IUDs. Individuals who are HIV-infected were also previously felt not to be appropriate candidates, but under certain circumstances the IUD may actually be found to be the best option for them. The end result of the listing of potential side effects and restricted user profiles, designed to protect against litigation, is to cause some health-care providers to avoid the provision of IUDs as a contraceptive option.

Women who have had a prior ectopic pregnancy are able to use a copper—but probably not a progesterone-bearing—IUD. On the other hand, women with excessive menstrual bleeding may actually be helped by the insertion of a Progestasert™.

Poor Candidates for IUD Use

Not all women are good candidates for the use of an IUD. Some have abnormalities such as multiple fibroids which distort the uterus; others have uterine cavities that are too small or too large. IUDs should not be inserted if there is any evidence of infection of the uterus, cervix, or vagina. Once an infection has been successfully treated, IUD insertion can proceed as planned. Any unexplained vaginal bleeding is a contraindication until the cause is found and dealt with appropriately; such bleeding could be due to such things as an undiagnosed pregnancy, acute or chronic PID, or an endocrine disorder. It is particularly important to investigate any suspicion of a genital malignancy, particularly in the presence of a highly abnormal Pap smear.

IUDs are not a good choice for a woman with severe uterine cramping (dysmenorrhea) because her symptoms may be accentuated by the presence of the device. Similarly, heavy menstrual bleeding should rule out the use of a copper-bearing IUD but may actually be an indication for one containing progesterone.

If a woman has multiple sexual partners or her partner or partners do, this places her at high risk for PID and makes her a poor candidate for intrauterine contraception.

There are a number of medical conditions that are usually listed as relative contraindications to IUD use. Among these are bacterial endocarditis, congenital or acquired valvular heart disease, leukemia, severe anemia, and sickle cell disease. Also the use of certain medications makes IUDs a poor choice, particularly anticoagulants which might lead to severe bleeding and chronic corticosteroid therapy, which carries an increased risk of infection.

Rarely, a woman will be found to have an allergy to copper and even more rarely, suffer from Wilson's disease, a congenital defect in copper excretion which is found in one out of every two hundred thousand women.

Instructions for Use

When a woman indicates an interest in using an IUD and is found to be a good candidate, her health-care provider should show her a device and tell her how it works and what to expect during the insertion procedure.

It is just as important, if not more so, to tell her what she may anticipate once she has been given an IUD. She should be told of any side effects that may develop, which are to be anticipated (requiring no medical care) and which are serious (requiring immediate medical intervention). If told what to expect in terms of temporary side effects, most women will usually tolerate them quite well. If not, many women react very badly to the symptoms that commonly occur shortly after insertion, which may lead them to ask prematurely for removal.

A woman must be warned that she may experience cramps for the first one to three days, and sometimes slightly longer. These are usually mild and easily treated with aspirin, ibuprofen, or naproxen. She should be aware of the fact that she may have slightly heavier bleeding with her next few menstrual periods and may temporarily experience intermenstrual bleeding or spotting. Finally, she must be warned that, although slight cramping and bleeding are common at first, if they continue or intensify she should return to her health-care provider for re-evaluation.

She also needs to know that it is essential that she check for the presence of the tail of her device at least after each menstrual period, and return for evaluation if she is unable to feel it, and that she should watch for expulsion. In either of these events, she should use a backup form of contraception, usually male latex condoms, until she sees her health-care provider. If she misses a menstrual period, she should be reevaluated promptly to see if she is pregnant.

It is important to discuss STDs with her and point out that her IUD will offer no protection against transmission of such diseases. If her sexual pattern changes and she has new partners, she must be urged to use male latex condoms in addition to her IUD. She must also be told about the signs and symptoms of pelvic infection and the importance of prompt medical treatment if they should occur.

She must know that she is protected against pregnancy right away after the insertion but that pregnancies, although rare, can occur, in the uterus and the fallopian tubes. She should be aware of the symptoms of ectopic pregnancy and of the extreme urgency for her to seek immediate medical attention should such symptoms develop.

Finally, she should know when to return for a new IUD, depending on the type that she is using, if she wishes to continue with this method of contraception. Nonmedicated IUDs such as the Lippes Loops may be used for as long as contraception is desired. As already noted, the ParaGard™ has at least a ten-year duration of use; the Progestasert™ must be changed annually. The removal procedure should be explained to her and she must know that her fertility will return as soon as her IUD is out.

A woman should be evaluated four to six weeks after insertion to make sure that there are no problems and to answer any questions she may have. After that, she should return for reevaluation at about one-year intervals (or earlier if she experiences any difficulties).

Myths and Misperceptions

Misinformation about the use of IUDs has had two very unfortunate outcomes in the United States: unnecessary fears and poor use.

One of the major deterrents to IUD acceptance is the misperception that they are very dangerous because they cause pelvic infections. Recent studies have shown that this is not the case, except for a slightly increased risk immediately after insertion. The myth is perpetuated by phenomena such as the disastrous experience with the Dalkon Shield and the current epidemics of STDs within the general population.

Of almost equal importance is the misperception that IUDs act by producing abortions. All of the current evidence points to the fact that IUDs act *prior* to fertilization by preventing the union of sperm with the egg.

Despite considerable evidence to the contrary, some people still believe that IUDs cause ectopic pregnancies and that babies born to women who become pregnant with their IUDs in place will be abnormal. There have also been concerns that copper coming off the IUDs could be toxic. This has never been an issue, however, because the measured daily release falls far below the amount of copper in the average diet.

Finally, the myth persists that IUDs cause sterility. Once again, there are no facts to support this fear. Most women can become pregnant shortly after their devices have been removed.

Usage

IUDs are the most frequently used long-term reversible contraceptives in the world. Unfortunately, they continue to be badly underutilized in the United States, primarily because of the multiple misunderstandings. For a while, the use of the plastic nonmedicated IUDs (the Lippes Loops and less often the Saf-T-Coil) was on the rise. However, their sales were discontinued in 1983 and 1985, respectively, for commercial reasons, when the medicated devices came onto the market and began to gain in popularity.

As already noted, the major controversy over the Dalkon Shield and its subsequent removal from the market in 1975, proved to be very destructive and, unfortunately, its impact is still being felt today. Many lawsuits resulted; some were justified and others were frivolous. These, in turn, led to hundreds of suits against the manufacturers of all other IUDs, many of the claims being totally unwarranted. These legal actions were very costly and soon made product liability insurance virtually unobtainable; they also brought research and development of new IUDs to an almost complete halt.

Because of the growing threat of litigation and the anticipated costs of defending hundreds of cases, G. D. Searle withdrew the Cu-7™ and Tatum-T™ on January 31, 1986. It did this despite the fact that both devices were still FDA-approved and that the company had won most of the lawsuits. This left the Progestasert™, made by Alza Pharmaceuticals, as the only IUD on the market for the next two years. However, as already noted, this device had never made a major impact on IUD usage. Within a few years, many women and even some health-care providers were unaware that IUDs were still available as a contraceptive option. As a result, the estimated number of IUD users dropped from 2.2 million in 1982 to 700,000 in 1988.

Then in 1988, the most effective of the copper-bearing IUDs, the ParaGard™ (TCu-380A), was finally introduced in the United States by GynoPharma, although it had been approved by the FDA several years earlier. Despite this, there has been no overall increase in the rate of utilization in recent years, and IUDs are now used by less than 1 percent of American women.

On the other hand, the worldwide use of IUDs has been increasing steadily. In the late 1970s, there were about 60 million women wearing IUDs, by 1978 there were approximately 84 million. Currently more than 128 million women are estimated to be using intrauterine contraception. The international rates of IUD usage vary widely from country to country. The devices are particularly popular in Asia, especially in China, which is using more than two-thirds of all of the IUDs employed today; 33 percent of all married Chinese women have IUDs. They are also quite popular in Scandinavia and Europe, where 18 percent or more of married women wear them. One or more of the copper-bearing IUDs are now being used in more than seventy developing countries.

There are several factors that contribute to the variability of IUD usage. Key among these are cultural differences. They are used most often in those countries where they are highly regarded by both women and their health-care providers. The availability of IUDs also varies considerably and depends, to a large degree, upon whether or not there are enough people skilled in IUD management. To deal with this problem, in many areas of the world nurses and other health-care workers have been successfully trained in the insertion and removal of IUDs and the care of women wearing these devices.

While the initial cost of an IUD and its insertion may sometimes prove to be a major deterrent, this factor is now beginning to be far less significant than the ones already outlined. The current pressures to provide effective contraception to women in the various health-care plans are gaining ground, particularly as there is a greater understanding of the cost-effectiveness of doing so as compared to the expenses incurred with unplanned pregnancies, both those carried to term and those terminated by induced abortions. At present, for insurance purposes, the IUD is considered to be a reversible contraceptive like the OCs, Norplant, and the diaphragm. Its use is covered by 39 percent of conventional plans, 50 percent of HMO plans, 44 percent of PPO plans, and 60 percent of POS plans. It is also covered by Medicaid in forty-six states and the District of Columbia.

There are two major reasons for the continued underutilization of IUDs in the United States, in contrast to the higher rates of usage seen in other countries. First, the very negative image of IUDs generated in the Dalkon Shield era, widely publicized in this country but less so in other parts of the world, unfortunately still persists. As a result, both health-care providers and their patients continue to shy away from IUDs unnecessarily. In addition, doctors are afraid of potential litigation, although there is no evidence that this need be a concern. To date, there have been no successful lawsuits brought against either the people doing the insertions or the manufacturers of the ParaGard™.

Second, IUD insertion is not being taught in many of the 272 residency training programs in obstetrics and gynecology in the United States. A recent survey revealed that one-third of chief (finishing) residents had never inserted an IUD, another third had inserted five or fewer, and only one-third had inserted more than five. As a result, they were not likely to use IUDs once they were in practice, nor would they include intrauterine contraception as part of future training curricula.

The importance of women's attitudes and where they get their information about IUDs has been pointed out very clearly in a number of recent surveys. In one study, IUDs had a low favorability rating—16 percent versus 76 percent for OCs. Interestingly enough, actual IUD users had the highest rating of satisfaction—99 percent versus 91 percent for OCs. It was also found that younger American women were more apt to select IUDs as their contraceptive method of choice than the older age group. Moreover, Hispanic women born outside the United States were noted to be more willing to use IUDs than those born in the United States; this suggests that they had had a lower level of exposure to adverse media reports. It also suggests that IUD usage could be considerably improved by both public and professional educational efforts.

In addition to the usual practice of interval IUD insertions, there are three other possible times for starting their use, all of which are even more underutilized. The first is following a first-trimester abortion, either spontaneous or induced; in the latter case, pregnancy is clearly not desired. In both situations, the woman is usually already in the health-care system. IUD insertions at this time have been demonstrated to be both safe and effective, and expulsion rates are very low.

Second, IUDs can also be inserted immediately following or shortly after a normal delivery, at a time when another pregnancy is also rarely desired immediately. The insertion is easy to do, the woman is already receiving medical care, and the added cost is low. Expulsion rates of immediate insertions are lower than those obtained when the insertions are delayed for several days. Special IUDs with long tails are used in these situations, and are trimmed at the postpartum visit.

Finally, IUDs provide an excellent form of emergency contraception, with a number of advantages over the hormonal methods. Estrogens, progestins, and OCs may be given for only up to seventy-two hours after unprotected intercourse whereas IUDs are effective for up to five days. Moreover, the nausea and vomiting often caused by hormone use are avoided. The failure rate of this use of IUDs is extremely low, 0.1 percent. Of even greater importance, the woman then has safe and effective long-term contraception, instead of protection for only a single event, if she elects to continue its use.

Future IUDs

A number of other IUDs are either under development or are being used in other countries. Research in this area has been aimed at finding devices that will be easier to insert and remove and have fewer side effects. Several of these—the Sof-T, the Fincoid-350, and the CuSafe 300—are basically T-shaped and contain copper. Another approach is an intracervical fixing device, which has a projection at the lower end that anchors the device in the endocervical canal. Finally, a very different device, the Gyne-Fix, has been studied for the past decade. It is made of semi-rigid suture material onto which six copper sleeves totaling 330 mm^2 of copper are threaded. The device is anchored to and suspended from the top of the uterine cavity by inserting a knot of the suture material at the end of the device into the uterine wall. Because it is small and flexible, this IUD produces less cramping and bleeding.

All of these devices are quite effective and can be used for a variable number of years. However, it is considered unlikely that any of them or any of the others under development will be introduced into the United States any time soon, with a single exception. This IUD, currently being used in ten other countries, is the levonorgestrel intrauterine system (LNG-IUS), also known as the Mirena™ or Levonova. It was approved in 1990 for use in Finland and it has been on the market there since 1991. It has been used by about 2 million women in Europe over the past decade. It was approved by the FDA on December 6, 2000, and is now available.

The design of the Mirena™ is similar to that of the Progestasert™, but it contains 52 mg of a different progestin, levonorgestrel; it releases 20 mcg a day. This device was originally developed because it was believed that the progestin would reduce uterine contractions that led to expulsions. It acts by thickening cervical mucus, inhibiting sperm motility, and altering the endometrium. It is approved for five years of use, and is highly effective, with a pregnancy rate of less than 1 percent. Protection starts as soon as the IUD is inserted; fertility is restored as soon as it is removed. Preliminary data suggest that it may also decrease the risk of PID. Its major difference from the copper devices lies in its effects on menstruation, reducing blood loss and even, on occasion, resulting in amenorrhea. This characteristic makes it of particular value to women who have iron-deficiency anemia or excessive menses. The Mirena™ may also have several additional uses—the treatment of dysfunctional uterine bleeding, fibroids, endometriosis, adenomyosis, endometrial hyperplasia, and pelvic inflammatory disease. It may be of particular value as part of hormone replacement therapy for postmenopausal women.

6

Female Barrier Contraceptives

BARRIER CONTRACEPTIVES, USED at the time of sexual intercourse, are among the oldest and most widely employed forms of birth control used by women. However, when the new methods whose use was unrelated to the time of sexual intercourse—OCs and IUDs—became available, these earlier techniques fell into relative disuse. Some of the older barrier methods are now regaining popularity and new ones are being studied. The primary reason for this is the growing concern about our rapidly rising rates of STDs, particularly incurable viral infections such as HIV/AIDS.

There are a number of good reasons for using barriers. First, they are very safe. Some women have medical contraindications to or do not wish to use other forms of family planning for personal reasons. For others, sexual intercourse may only be sporadic and they see no need for the continuous use of other methods, which they often regard as being potentially dangerous. Second, a woman can use barrier contraceptives while waiting to have a tubal ligation, to start OCs, or to have an IUD inserted or between methods or as a back-up method for missed pills and lost IUDs. Third, some women elect to use barriers only at midcycle, at the time of presumed ovulation. Finally, there are those who find that their access to health care is very limited or they prefer, for one of any number of reasons, not to get into the health-care system.

While all of these reasons are important, in addition to the avoidance of unwanted pregnancies the greatest impetus for the use of barriers today is to prevent STD transmission. Many of these diseases have reached epidemic and even pandemic proportions and have led to millions of infections and deaths. These infections include chlamydia, syphilis, gonorrhea, herpes, cytomegalovirus, human papillomavirus (HPV), and, especially, human immunodeficiency virus (HIV).

One of the biggest public health concerns today is the transmission of HIV/AIDS. This is particularly important to women as they are up to seventeen times more likely to become infected by an HIV-positive male partner than vice versa. The evidence is now very clear that the use of barriers, particularly the latex male condom, provides significant protection against the spread of HIV.

Currently, studies are being carried out on both old and new barrier methods to determine how well they protect against STD transmission. Early data have already shown that the risks related to STDS and PID can be reduced, at least by half, with the proper and consistent use of barrier contraceptives. This, in turn, will lower the risks of infertility and ectopic pregnancy, both of which are usually the direct result of these infections.

A final reason, although less commonly a key consideration, is the fact that barrier methods can help to protect against the development of cervical cancer by blocking HPV infections, currently believed to be the major cause of this malignancy. It is now well established that women who have never used barrier contraceptives are almost twice as apt to develop this disease as women who have.

When a woman elects to use a barrier method, her health-care provider must inform her that it is absolutely essential that she use it each time she has intercourse. Diaphragms and cervical caps must be properly fitted and women must be taught how to insert, remove and take care of them. Other barriers do not require a medical visit, and can be purchased over the counter. In either case, a woman must read the instructions very carefully for the particular method that she is going to use and keep them for future review. Finally, no matter which barrier method is used, she should not douche for six hours after intercourse.

Spermicides

Spermicides prevent pregnancy by exerting a destructive chemical action on the membrane covering the head of the sperm. This chemical renders the sperm incapable of fertilizing an egg. The membrane becomes more permeable, the intracellular material leaks out, and the sperm lose their mobility. The most commonly used agent is nonoxynol-9 (N9). It is a surfactant (surface-active agent) found also in dish soaps, where it acts to break up food particles, especially fat, an effect similar to that which makes it useful as a contraceptive.

Spermicides also act in the same fashion on some of the organisms that cause STDs, destroying them or blocking their growth. Laboratory studies have shown that N9 will inhibit the growth of gonorrhea, candida, trichomoniasis, and the herpes virus; clinical studies, although relatively small and few in number, have suggested a lower incidence of these diseases in women using spermicides. The search to find even more potent anti-infective products (microbicides) continues.

Description

There are several ways to deliver spermicides into the vagina, e.g., jellies, creams, foams, foaming tablets, and foaming and melting suppositories. Most of these products contain one of three chemicals—either N9 or, less often, octoxynol or menfegol. The active agent is mixed into a vehicle which is chemically inert; its primary function is to carry and then release the spermicide.

Another method of dispersing a spermicide is to place it in a film. Such a product has been used in Europe for many years, where it has been known as C-film. It is now sold in the United States as VCF (Vaginal Contraceptive Film). It must be placed high in the vagina about five minutes prior to intercourse, where it melts, releasing a spermicide adequate for two hours of protection. Its only side effect is local irritation, and its effectiveness is generally comparable to that of the other barrier methods.

In the foam preparations, foaming agents and propellants are added to the spermicide. It is believed that the vehicle in these products may possibly increase the effectiveness of the spermicide by coating the upper vagina and blocking the cervix, acting as a mechanical barrier. Spermicides are also used with the male condom as added protection against both pregnancy and STD transmission.

Effectiveness

No major differences in effectiveness have been found in formal studies conducted on the various barrier methods, but there is considerable variation in the effectiveness rates obtained with the general use of these products. They can be as high as 97 percent with perfect use, but usually average about 79 percent; however, some studies have reported rates that are considerably lower with inconsistent use. Clearly, no other contraceptive category has such a wide range of values for effectiveness, which illustrates how lapses in compliance can negatively affect a method's overall ability to prevent unwanted pregnancies.

Usage

To use barrier contraceptives most effectively women need to follow the instructions for each type of spermicide. Foaming products must be shaken vigorously before being put into their applicators. It is important to place creams, jellies, and foaming products high in the vagina so that the cervix is covered. Creams and jellies need a few minutes to melt, but foams are almost instantly dispersed. If an hour elapses before intercourse, a second application of the spermicide should be made. Similarly, it should be repeated with each subsequent act of intercourse. If tablets, suppositories, or film are used, women must be sure to wait the indicated length of time so that adequate amounts of the spermicide are released.

Safety

In December 1980, the FDA issued a report from its Panel on Vaginal Contraceptives. It contained an extensive review of all of the ingredients in these products, classifying them into three categories—safe and effective (I), not safe and/or not effective (II), and data inadequate to make a determination (III). Category I ingredients were allowed to stay on the market, Category II ingredients had to be removed, and Category III ingredients had to have additional study data submitted to the FDA before they could be approved for use. Category I included the three ingredients already mentioned. Mercury-containing products were placed in Category II because of known adverse effects on animal embryos. Mercury had also been found to produce severe damage in humans in Japan—Minamata's disease—as a result of consumption of fish containing toxic levels of mercury. As a side note, the FDA has issued a new warning that pregnant women should avoid certain fish because of their high mercury content.

In addition to classifying all of the ingredients, the panel also recommended a screening process for testing during the development of new vaginal contraceptives. It included extensive animal studies, looking for toxicity in both adults and fetuses, and also at pregnancy outcomes. Laboratory testing for chromosomal damage and tumor induction were to be carried out in cell cultures. All of these were to be completed prior to the start of any evaluations in the human.

There has been considerable medical and legal controversy in recent years as to whether or not spermicides are safe. The problems began when a badly flawed study was published in 1981, which suggested that certain congenital abnormalities (including limb-reduction defects, chromosomal changes, and tumors) could be linked to the mother's use of a spermicide at the time of conception. However, the use of the spermicide was only presumed, since to become a subject in the study, a woman need only to have filled a prescription for one within six hundred days of the birth of the baby. It was never determined when it was used in the course of the pregnancy, or, in fact, whether it was used at all.

A widely celebrated lawsuit resulted from this article. When a $5,151,030 judgment was rendered in favor of the plaintiff, there was serious concern that spermicides might fall prey to a new round of litigation frenzy. Fortunately, this did not occur; numerous studies, reported both before and after the trial, have clearly shown no adverse effects with the use of spermicidal agents and they are not currently labeled with any such warning.

The only problem noted with most of the spermicidal agents is a 2 to 4 percent incidence of local sensitivity on the part of either the male and/or the female. A sensation of heat and burning has been noted, particularly with foaming suppositories. (Interestingly, this is reportedly pleasurable to some users.)

Advantages

Spermicides offer several advantages. When used properly and consistently their effectiveness rates are relatively high, although not reaching the levels achieved by IUDs and the hormonal methods. They are widely available over-the-counter in retail stores, outlets, and pharmacies. No medical intervention is required, no prescription is needed, and confidentiality is usually maintained. Moreover, their cost is low and they have a long shelf life; they may be kept on hand for intermittent use for a considerable length of time.

There is another advantage to the use of spermicides for a particular group of women. These are the individuals who suffer from vaginal dryness, especially those approaching menopause whose estrogen levels are dropping. The lubricating effect of spermicides is often of considerable benefit in this situation.

Disadvantages

Barrier methods are not the right choice for some women. Those who have very strong personal or medical contraindications to pregnancy should be advised that barrier contraceptives are not, in general, as effective as the hormonal methods and IUDs. Many women (and men) are unwilling to use a technique that, to be effective, must be used correctly with each act of intercourse. In addition, careful attention must be given to the time required for the spermicide to become effective in the various products. Moreover, some people find the need to repeat spermicide use with each act of intercourse annoying.

Some women complain that barrier methods are messy; they dislike the excess fluid and leakage these contraceptives produce. Some also find the odor of the spermicide offensive. Finally, in certain cultures women are taught not to touch their genital organs; barriers, therefore, are not appropriate options for these individuals.

Diaphragm

Prior to the development of hormonal contraceptives and IUDs, diaphragms were the most commonly used form of medical contraception in the United States. They declined sharply in popularity but are now being used again partly because of many fears, often unfounded, about the side effects of OCs and IUDs and also because of the recognition that they will protect, at least to some degree, against the transmission of STDs. For example, use of the diaphragm has been shown to cut the risk of acquiring PID in half; protection against certain STDs, including trichomoniasis and bacterial vaginosis, has also been documented.

Description

There are three major types of diaphragms—coil spring, flat metal spring, and arcing spring—each with its own particular advantages. Diaphragms are made in different sizes, measuring 50 to 105 mm in diameter; those between 65 and 80 mm are the most commonly used. They act as a physical barrier, covering the cervix and also as a vehicle for delivering a spermicide. Some women have found it difficult to insert the coil and flat metal spring diaphragms. Moreover, they should only be used by women with normal vaginal anatomy. The arching spring diaphragms are the easiest to insert and are the ones most often prescribed. Also, they can be used by women with poor vaginal muscle tone resulting in cystoceles and rectoceles.

Two other types of diaphragms are being studied. The first is the Lea Shield. It has a one-way flutter valve that prevents air from being trapped between it and the cervix during insertion and allows cervical secretions to escape. There is also a loop attached to the edge of the cap, which helps during insertion and removal. The FDA has refused approval of this device until larger clinical trials are completed. The second is the SILCS. It has a projection on one side and a dimpled surface, which make insertion and removal easier. The cost of this device is expected to be less than that of the standard diaphragm.

Effectiveness

The currently accepted effectiveness rates for the diaphragm used with a spermicidal cream or jelly are up to 97 percent with perfect use, but only 82 percent with average use. The added protection that comes with the simultaneous use of male condoms raises their combined effectiveness a bit closer to that of the other more effective methods.

As with all other barrier methods, the level of effectiveness of the diaphragm is enhanced by good instruction along with proper and consistent use.

Usage

Diaphragms must be prescribed by a trained health worker who will first check for any contraindications to the use of this method. The proper size is determined by using sterile fitting rings of various diameters. It is important that diaphragms be fitted properly. If too small a device is used, it may not cover the cervix properly and pregnancy may result. If it is too large, it may be uncomfortable to either the woman or her sexual partner and may be displaced. Some researchers have suggested that pressure on the urethra by a diaphragm that is too large may possibly cause acute or chronic urinary tract infections, but this has never been totally proved.

A woman must learn what her cervix feels like with and without the diaphragm in place. After the proper size has been determined, the woman should practice inserting and removing the diaphragm, initially in the clinic or doctor's office and then at home. After about a week, she should return for a checkup to make sure that she is putting the diaphragm in properly and to ask for any additional information to ensure correct usage.

The diaphragm may be inserted either immediately or up to six hours before intercourse. A teaspoonful of spermicide must be placed in the dome of the diaphragm which goes over the cervix. Spermicide should also be spread around the rim and the outside surface of the dome. After a woman places her diaphragm in her vagina, she must check for its proper position; it should completely cover the cervix.

A diaphragm must be left in place for six hours after sexual relations. If intercourse occurs again within this time frame, additional spermicide must be put in the vagina without removing the diaphragm and another six hours allowed to elapse. A diaphragm should not be left in the vagina for longer than twenty-four hours. A woman must take care not to damage the diaphragm during removal; long fingernails can be particularly dangerous. To remove the diaphragm the woman should insert her index finger under the rim of the diaphragm to break the suction and then gently pull it out. Following removal, it must be carefully checked for holes, washed with warm water and mild unscented soap, sprinkled with unscented talcum powder or corn starch and stored in a dark cool place. Diaphragms should be rechecked and replaced every two years. They should also be rechecked after a pregnancy to be sure that they still fit properly.

Safety

There are no consistently reported significant side effects to the use of the diaphragm, other than the questionable effect on urinary tract infections and a 2 to 4 percent sensitivity to the latex rubber or to the spermicide. Minor erosions of the vaginal walls have been noted occasionally; these are caused by the pressure of the rim of the diaphragm. What role this may play in vaginal infections remains unclear.

Recently, questions have been raised about the possible association between diaphragm use and toxic shock syndrome (TSS). These cases were rare and were most often seen in women who left their diaphragms in place for longer than twenty-four hours, giving rise to the speculation that this encouraged the growth of bacteria in the vagina.

Advantages

The diaphragm is attractive to women who are concerned about the safety of IUDs and hormonal methods. If they follow instructions conscientiously, they can achieve quite a high level of effectiveness, particularly if accompanied by the use of the male latex condom. As noted, diaphragms may be inserted hours before intercourse.

Disadvantages

Medical intervention is required in order to use a diaphragm. To be effective, it must be used every time a woman has sexual relations. The diaphragm must be properly inserted, removed, inspected, and stored, all of which require some degree of privacy. Some women dislike the messiness of the spermicide and the need to use an additional amount for repeated acts of intercourse. Others object to having to leave it in place for six hours after use. Women with marked degrees of pelvic relaxation cannot use this method.

Finally, poor levels of motivation, as determined by prior performance, should suggest that this may not be the best option for certain women.

Cervical Cap

The first cervical cap was made in 1838 by a German gynecologist. He fashioned a wax mold of the cervix of each patient requesting this device and then produced a cap for that particular woman. A similar approach was tried in the United States in the late 1980s, but both attempts proved to be unsuccessful.

The cervical cap was used for a number of years in the United States, Britain, and Europe in the early and mid-1900s prior to the advent of hormone contraceptives and IUDs. Then, for a considerable number of years, a cervical cap was not available in the United States. However, when there was renewed interest in this type of contraception, a number of studies were undertaken on three caps, all made of rubber.

Description

The Vimule cap was bell-shaped, had a flanged rim, and was made in three sizes: 42, 48, and 54 mm. It covered the cervix and the upper part of the vagina and was held in place by its rim. It was designed for use by women with long cervices. The rubber used was very firm and it turned out that its rim caused lacerations; as a consequence, research on this cap was discontinued.

Another cap that was investigated was the Dumas cap. It was shallow and bowl-shaped, and it too covered both the cervix and upper vagina. It was made in five sizes, ranging from 50 to 75 mm. It was used in women who had a short cervix. However, there was never sufficient interest in this product to bring it to the marketplace.

A third cap, the Prentif Cavity Rim Cervical Cap™, was thimble-shaped. It covered only the cervix and was held in place by suction. It was made in four sizes: 22, 25, 28, and 31 mm. It was designed for the average size cervix. The diameter of the cap had to be slightly smaller than the base of the cervix so that it touched the vaginal walls.

The various studies resulted in the introduction of only one of the caps, the Prentif Cap. It was marketed after being approved by the FDA in 1988, and it is still available today.

Another cap, the FemCap, is currently being evaluated. Early evidence suggests that it may be easier to fit and use and may be somewhat more effective. It has a strap on the bottom to help in removal. The FemCap is made of nonallergic silicone rubber, which removes the potential problem of latex allergy.

Effectiveness

The cervical cap has about the same level of effectiveness as the diaphragm. It acts both as a mechanical barrier and as a chemical barrier by the addition of a spermicide. Unlike the diaphragm, most caps cover only the cervix and not the entire upper vagina. They are held in place by suction, not a spring. Only rarely are they dislodged during sexual intercourse or felt by the male. As with other barrier methods, the effectiveness of the cap is directly related to how well and consistently it is used.

Usage

Like the diaphragm, a cap must be carefully fitted by people trained in this procedure. They need to first examine the cervix to see if the woman is an appropriate candidate. The cap is contraindicated for women with certain structural abnormalities and for those with infections of the cervix. However, caps may sometimes be used by women who have anatomical contraindications to the use of a diaphragm such as marked pelvic relaxation resulting in cystoceles, rectoceles, and uterine prolapse.

Despite the fact that the Prentif Caps come in four sizes, only about 80 percent of the patients who want a cap can be properly fitted with the ones that are currently available. Also, it takes between half an hour to an hour to teach the average woman to use this method and some find it difficult or impossible to learn. A woman must be able to identify her cervix and to know how it feels with the cap over it.

The cap may be used alone or, at the time of insertion, it may be half filled with spermicide, which will increase its overall effectiveness up to a failure rate of only 6 percent. The spermicide will also help to decrease the problem of vaginal discharge and odor that some women experience after twenty-four hours of use. Although the cap may be left in place for one or two days and used with repeated acts of intercourse without added spermicide, the position must be checked each time to be sure that it is still properly in place over the cervix. To make sure that no viable sperm are left in the vagina, the cap must be left in for at least eight hours after the last instance of intercourse.

To remove the cap, it should be tipped to break the seal and then it can be hooked with the index finger and pulled out gently. Caring for the cap is similar to caring for a diaphragm. Difficulty in reaching the cervix is often overcome by squatting or bearing down, which will bring the cervix lower in the vagina.

Caps are well accepted by certain women. Others who have attempted to use them complain of problems in insertion and removal. Caps are more difficult to insert than diaphragms and must be placed directly over the cervix. In general, the continuation rates have not been very good; many women discontinue use of their caps within a year.

Safety

There are no serious adverse effects from the use of the cap other than occasional sensitivity to the latex or the added spermicide. There are no reports linking TSS to the use of caps. Although there is a theoretical potential for the growth of bacteria inside the cap, no pelvic infections have been reported.

Advantages

The major advantages of the caps are their safety and the fact that they can be inserted at a time unrelated to intercourse and may be left in place for one to two days. They do not need to be used with a spermicide, but this may be desirable as already noted, although it adds to the expense involved. However, less spermicide is required and so caps are perceived as less messy. Although it has not yet been proved, using a cap may help to prevent the spread of STDs and HIV/AIDS. This is because the cap covers the cervix, which is now believed to be the principal site of transmission of these diseases.

Disadvantages

Disadvantages to cap use are the fact that they require medical intervention since they come in several sizes, and that not all women are good candidates for this form of birth control. Women with a cervix that is too short or too long cannot use the cap, and not all women can be fitted. They are sometimes dislodged during intercourse. Satisfaction rates tend to be fairly low and discontinuation rates are often high.

Vaginal Contraceptive Sponge

The use of sponges in the vagina to prevent pregnancy goes back in time as far as the ancient Egyptians. Once women connected sexual intercourse with pregnancy, they gathered sponges from the ocean and cut them into pieces, which they placed in their vaginas prior to coitus.

Over the years attempts have been made to develop modern versions of the ancient sea sponges. A wide variety of materials has been tried, initially without conspicuous success. In the mid-1970s sponges made out of collagen were studied but they were large, rough and unattractive and never brought to the marketplace.

Several other types of sponges were developed and tested. However, only one underwent sufficient laboratory and clinical testing, over a period of seven years, to meet the requirements for submission to the FDA. A formal presentation was made by the manufacturer, the VLI Corporation, to the FDA's medical advisory committee on October 28, 1982. When the committee reviewed the device, it recommended that the sponge be approved for forty-eight hours of use. In fact the company had planned to name it the "2 Day Sponge." The FDA, however, disagreed and restricted its duration of use to twenty-four hours, so it became the Today Sponge™.

After approval for marketing was given by the FDA in March of 1983, the sponge was widely distributed and used, becoming the most popular over-the-counter vaginal contraceptive method. By 1995, the contraceptive sponge had more than 115,000 users.

In 1987, the sponge was sold to Whitehall Robbins Healthcare, a division of American Home Products. It manufactured the sponge until 1995 when it voluntarily halted production. The FDA had recently established more stringent manufacturing requirements and questioned the purity of the air and water at the plant where the sponges were made. Since meeting these new FDA requirements would have been very expensive, it was decided to cease production and close the plant. There was no concern about the safety of the sponge, and it is still approved by the FDA; however, no sponges have been available in the United States since that time.

The Allendale Company, which now owns the sponge, is seeking FDA approval to reenter the market. It is widely believed that this will occur quite soon. The company made a presentation to the FDA on July 12, 2000 and is continuing to work with it to complete the additional requirements outlined by the FDA. The return of the sponge will be applauded by many women, particularly those in the younger age group, for many of whom it was the contraceptive method of choice.

Description

The Vaginal Contraceptive Sponge is made of polyurethane and is produced in a single size, 55 mm in diameter and 30 mm in thickness. The sponge is shaped like a mushroom and the concave side is placed over the cervix. It is soft, disposable, and has a polyester loop attached to the bottom of the device to facilitate removal. It contains 1 gm of N9 and releases 125–150 mg in twenty-four hours. This is 10 to 20 percent of the total amount and is less than that released from some other vaginal contraceptives, particularly if multiple applications are made for repeated acts of sexual intercourse within a period of several hours.

Two other sponges are available in other countries. The Protectaid™ sponge contains N9, benzalkonium chloride (BZK), and sodium cholate. It has been marketed in Canada since 1966 and is now approved for use in Europe. The Pharmatex™ sponge contains 60 mg of BZK. It is being marketed in Europe. A third sponge, the Avert™ sponge, uses N9 and is under investigation. All three of these sponges are made in only one size and are sold over the counter. The instructions for their use are similar to those for the Today Sponge. One of the added advantages of the Protectaid and Avert sponges is the fact that they are already wet when purchased, so no water needs to be added before insertion.

Effectiveness

The effectiveness rates of the Today Sponge have been widely debated because of differences noted in some studies between women who had and had not borne children. They ranged from 72 to 92 percent for the first group, and 82 to 95 percent for the second. Sponges are generally believed to be slightly more effective than spermicides but slightly less effective than the diaphragm and the male latex condom.

Usage

The Today Sponge acts in three ways: by slowly releasing N9 into the vagina, by blocking the cervix, and by absorbing semen and trapping the sperm and exposing them to the N9.

The sponge is moistened with water, squeezed to remove any extra fluid, and inserted over the cervix at any time up to twenty-four hours prior to intercourse. It may be used immediately and remains effective for twenty-four hours for multiple acts of intercourse without adding additional spermicide. It should be left in place for six hours after the last coitus and is removed by pulling on the loop. Many women find the sponge less messy and easier to use than other forms of vaginal contraception.

Safety

No serious side effects were found during clinical testing of the sponge. One of the ongoing concerns raised about sponge use has been the possible induction of the toxic shock syndrome. Cases of TSS began to be reported in the late 1970s, primarily in healthy young women who were users of high-absorbency menstrual tampons. It was found to be caused by a particular bacteria, staphylococcus aureus. Subsequently, this disease was also found to occur in non-menstruating women, children, and men. Individuals suffering from TSS have nausea, vomiting and diarrhea, a high fever that comes on suddenly, hypotension, muscle pain, and damage to the liver, kidneys, and brain. A diffuse skin rash appears and, after about one to two weeks, desquamation (shedding) of the skin of the palms of the hands and the soles of the feet begins. The mortality rate runs between 3 to 13 percent.

Although no cases of TSS were found in the clinical trials involving 1,847 women and none have been reported with the proper use of the sponge, women are warned in the package insert about the symptoms of TSS and told not to use the sponge during their menstrual periods or after childbirth, since blood supports the growth of bacteria. Actually N9 appears, in laboratory testing, to be toxic to the organism that causes TSS.

Questions were raised in the past about the possible induction of malignancies by the use of the sponge. Multiple studies in rats, rabbits, and dogs have failed to reveal any potential for the development of any type of cancer. Even more important, widespread use of the sponge by several million women for more than twenty years has indicated no evidence of risk.

The sponge has been shown to produce vaginal irritation in about 1 to 4 percent of users, presumably due to N9; a similar incidence of sensitivity has been found in sexual partners. About 8 percent of users have complained of vaginal itching, soreness, or dryness. In comparative clinical trials, the sponge has been shown to produce less vaginal irritation than those products that use foaming and effervescent vehicles for the introduction of spermicides into the vagina. Moreover, one sponge may be used up to thirty hours, whereas all other vaginal spermicidal agents require additional applications for repeated acts of intercourse.

Advantages

The vaginal contraceptive sponge offers consumers a number of advantages. It is available over the counter and comes in only one size so that fitting is not required. It is easy to insert and may be placed in the vagina immediately before or up to twenty-four hours prior to intercourse. The sponge is effective for twenty-four to thirty hours after insertion for multiple acts of sexual intercourse without the need to add more spermicide. It has minimal side effects, is less messy than other vaginal barrier methods, and is disposable. Finally, it may protect against the transmission of certain STDs.

Disadvantages

The sponge is less effective than the IUD and hormonal contraceptives. To achieve maximum protection, the sponge must be properly inserted and be in the proper place with every act of intercourse, which requires a high level of compliance. The sponge may occasionally cause discomfort to one or both sexual partners; 1 to 4 percent of both men and women have been found to be sensitive to N9. There have been problems with removal of the sponge, particularly for new users. Finally, leaving the sponge in place for longer than the recommended time may cause a malodorous vaginal discharge.

Female Condom

The newest female barrier method to become available is the vaginal pouch, marketed as the Reality Female Condom™. It is the first method studied and approved under a protocol devised by the FDA to provide expedited fast-track approval for any technique with significant protection against both unwanted pregnancy and STD transmission. It is also the first condom that is controlled by the female. The FDA granted approval for marketing in 1993. However, it required the manufacturer to put a statement in the labeling that use of the male latex condom is the method of choice to prevent the transmission of STDs.

The female condom, also known as the contraceptive vaginal pouch, is also available in the United Kingdom and a number of other countries, primarily in Europe.

Description

The vaginal pouch is a polyurethane sheath about 17 cm long. The main portion of the sheath lines the entire vagina. The end which goes into the vagina is closed and covers the cervix. It is held in place by a flexible ring, rather like a diaphragm. The outer end, which is open, has a ring that covers part of the vulva and prevents contact with the base of the penis and the ejaculate.

Effectiveness

The vaginal pouch has failure rates that are comparable to those of other barrier methods. Clinical studies carried out on eighty-one women in the United States and Latin America reported a failure rate of 15.1 per one hundred women in the first six months of use.

Usage

The pouch is prelubricated with silicone, and it comes with a water-soluble lubricant. It may be inserted just before or several hours prior to coitus. The female condom is made in one size only and is sold over the counter. It is meant for single use, and it is disposable.

The wall of the pouch is about twice as thick as that of the male latex condoms. Polyurethane has been found to be less permeable than latex, and in laboratory testing, the passage of dyes, gases, HIV, trichomonads, and other organisms has been found to be blocked by this material. The clinical data on the female condom and the prevention of STD transmission are limited but one study did show a decreased incidence of trichomoniasis. However, as yet, no similar studies have been reported on the prevention of the transmission of other STD organisms although it has been estimated that if the device were used correctly with each act of intercourse that it could provide up to 94 percent protection.

Safety

No adverse effects have been found with the use of the pouch, either in the clinical trials or after general distribution following FDA approval in 1993.

Advantages

The major advantages of the female condom are its availability over the counter and the fact that it is controlled by the woman. It is an excellent alternative should the male partner refuse to wear a condom. The female condom also provides a significant degree of protection to the male, since the pouch is designed to cover the cervix, vagina, and part of the perineum. For the woman, it provides maximum protection against both sperm and infecting organisms.

Disadvantages

The major disadvantage of the pouch is aesthetic, its appearance being somewhat forbidding to both men and women. Also there have been reports of some problems in usage, such as the penis displacing the outer ring or entering the vagina outside the sheath. Finally, both men and women have complained that the devices are "noisy" during use.

7

Periodic Abstinence

THIS APPROACH TO CONTRACEPTION, previously known as rhythm and natural family planning, is of relatively recent origin inasmuch as it is based on a better understanding of the various factors involved in human reproduction, resulting from modern research. It operates on the premise that sexual intercourse must be avoided during the time each month when a woman can become pregnant. It is the only method of birth control acceptable to certain individuals and religious groups. Whereas it was used quite often prior to the introduction of the OCs and IUDs, a study in 1988 showed that it was used by only about 1 percent of American women at that time.

Several centuries ago, people began to try to determine the patterns of fertility and, somewhat later, the accurate detection of the fertile period. In recent years, the ability to measure the various hormonal levels in women has led to a more accurate and detailed description of the normal menstrual cycle. Although it was clear to our ancestors that pregnancy was related to sexual intercourse, the exact way in which it came about was unknown until 1677 when Antonie van Leeuwenhoek first looked through his microscope and saw active sperm in human seminal fluid. Today, using highly specialized photographic equipment, it is actually possible to record ovulation and fertilization.

Many studies have looked into the duration of viability of both the egg and the sperm. It has been found that an egg can only be fertilized for approximately the first twelve to twenty-four hours after it is released from the ovary. Sperm, on the other hand, are viable for about forty-eight hours, and, on occasion, they have been shown to live for up to seven days when they were stored in the crypts of the endocervical canal and subsequently released. Finally, other studies have documented two additional important facts—first, that regardless of the length of a menstrual cycle, ovulation almost always occurs approximately fourteen days before the onset of the menstrual flow and, second, that the period of highest fertility is the day of ovulation and the two days before.

Methods

The Calendar Method

The calendar method was developed by following the length of a woman's menstrual cycles over a period of several months to determine the probable time of ovulation. In the 1930s, Knaus in Austria and Ogino in Japan studied the patterns of women's menstrual cycles. The length of the periods of fertility which they postulated were five days and eight days, respectively.

Prior to starting this method, the fertile period is determined in three steps. First, the shortest and longest cycles must be identified over a period of approximately six to twelve months. Second, the calculation of the first day of assumed fertility is done using the shortest recorded cycle minus eighteen days. Third, the calculation of the last day of the probable fertile period is done using the longest cycle minus eleven days.

Because many women have cycles that are slightly or markedly irregular, it is obvious that their required number of days of abstinence can be very high. For example, a woman who has recorded cycles going from twenty-six to thirty-two days must not have intercourse from the eighth to the twenty-first day of her cycle. This approach has been found to put considerable stress on couples and therefore, as would be expected, the continuation rates are quite low and the pregnancy rates are quite high.

The Temperature Method

Other methods of detecting the fertile period have been attempted over the years. One of the oldest of these is the temperature method. This technique is based on the observation that the basal body temperature (BBT) is elevated by 0.4 to 0.8 degrees F following ovulation, due to the production of progesterone by the ovary. It then remains elevated until the next menstrual period begins. Intercourse is not allowed from the time the menses stop until three days after the temperature rise occurs.

This method has several disadvantages. First, a woman using this technique must take her temperature every day before she gets out of bed and write it down. Second, other factors including infections and certain drugs can influence the temperature readings, making the accurate prediction of ovulation very problematic. Moreover, this technique, like the calendar method, requires couples to remain abstinent for considerable lengths of time.

The Cervical Mucus Method

More recently, studies have been carried out using the Billings method, which is based on the detection of certain changes in a woman's cervical mucus. The character of the mucus varies throughout the menstrual cycle, being thick, sticky, gray, and opaque except at the time of ovulation when it is thin, clear, and stringy which makes it receptive to the passage of sperm.

This technique was described by the Drs. E. L. and J. J. Billings of Australia in the 1970s. A woman using this method must check her cervical mucus daily. When it becomes more profuse, wet, slippery, and transparent and reaches a peak, it is presumed that the woman is ovulating. Intercourse is allowed during the dry days that follow the menstrual period. However, coitus should not take place on two consecutive days, since seminal fluid may prevent the detection of changes in the cervical mucus. Once mucus suggesting ovulation appears, then abstinence must be practiced until the fourth day after the peak.

This method has several noted advantages over the calendar and temperature methods. First, it does not require the measurement and daily recording of the BBT. Second, it permits a woman who has irregular cycles to have fewer days when she must abstain from sexual intercourse. However, the accuracy of the detection of cervical mucus changes may be quite difficult if a women has a vaginal discharge or is using vaginal medication or lubricants.

The Symptothermal Method

One of the most effective ways to use the periodic abstinence method requires a combination of the temperature method along with the identification of certain physical changes associated with the approach of ovulation and also the detection of cervical mucus changes. Women can be taught to look for certain symptoms and signs that indicate the likelihood that ovulation will occur in a few days. These include such things as enlargement and tenderness of the breasts, low back pain, pelvic pain (*mittelschmerz*), abdominal cramping and bloating, vulvar swelling, and mild vaginal bleeding or spotting. In addition, they can often detect a gradual softening of the cervix on self examination.

Use of the symptothermal method requires that women stop having intercourse when their BBT goes up and they develop symptoms and observe vaginal wetness and midcycle cervical mucus changes. They must abstain until the third day after the temperature rise or, alternatively, the fourth day after the cervical mucus has reached its peak. However, this approach has the same disadvantages as the ones already noted for both the temperature and cervical mucus detection methods.

Congenital Anomalies

A number of papers were published over a period of years suggesting that use of these techniques would increase the number of congenital abnormalities in babies conceived while periodic abstinence was being practiced. Earlier, it had been shown in animals that fertilization of older eggs produced chromosomal abnormalities, fetal deaths, and a higher rate of congenitally malformed offspring. The human studies that caused concern suggested that there was an increased incidence of spontaneous abortions, chromosomal abnormalities, and certain birth defects including cleft lip and palate, hydrocele, mental retardation, and Down's syndrome. However, the number of subjects in these studies was small, and there was considerable question as to the accuracy of the data since it was based on recalled information, which often contains considerable bias. A large WHO study on this subject did not show any increase in these problems, nor did it find that more male babies were conceived at the end of the fertile period than females, as had also been suggested.

Effectiveness

There is a very large difference in pregnancy rates obtained with the various forms of ovulation detection and periodic abstinence. The calendar method, used alone, has a pregnancy rate of about 40 percent. The temperature method, used alone, has pregnancy rates that vary from 0.3 to 6.6 percent; a couples can attain a very low rate if they adhere carefully to all the rules. Reported rates from the use of the cervical mucus method range from 5.3 to 32 percent.

The effectiveness of the symptothermal method has also been highly variable, according to WHO studies, going from a 17.7 percent failure rate in Dublin to 31 percent in Auckland. In general, pregnancy rates have ranged between 4.9 and 34.4 percent with an average of 15 percent. However, close adherence to all the recommendations can result in rates as low as 2 percent. Consistently high levels of effectiveness have been found when barrier methods—spermicides or condoms—are used during the fertile period.

Determinations of pregnancy rates in women using some form of periodic abstinence have been carried out in many countries and also in different population groups living in the same geographical area. They have been shown to have major differences. For example, the WHO's Task Force on Methods for the Determination of the Fertile Period followed 725 couples in five countries—El Salvador, India, Ireland, New Zealand, and the Philippines. It calculated that the failure rates in these programs varied from 3.1 to 86.4 percent.

The most successful natural family planning program that WHO found was in Mauritius. However, it was noted that a considerable amount of training time was required and many follow-up visits were made, as often as one to two times a week for the first three cycles and then once a week or up to three or four times a year thereafter. All of these studies made it very clear that the degree of success was highly dependent upon the quality of the instruction that the couples received and how well they were willing to adhere to it.

Over the years, a number of electronic, chemical, and mechanical ovulation-detecting techniques have been developed to try to make periodic abstinence more precise, easier to use, and thus more acceptable. The success of these techniques has been variable; some are fairly accurate, others less so, and still others rather expensive and too complicated for the average woman to use.

Advantages

As a birth control method, periodic abstinence has several advantages. First, it is safe (excluding the risks of pregnancy in the event of failure) and always available. Second, no drugs or devices are used that have side effects and thus are considered to be unnatural by some people. Third, the methods are relatively to highly effective if they are strictly adhered to, particularly if several methods are used concurrently. Fourth, there is minimal or no cost involved. Finally, it is acceptable to certain groups for whom other contraception methods are not.

Disadvantages

Periodic abstinence requires a very high level of motivation and constant commitment on the part of both the man and the woman. Since there is often considerable interference with sexual spontaneity and frequency, male partners may not always wish to cooperate. On the other hand, some successful users of this method have reported that the quality of their marriages has actually been improved by their use of periodic abstinence.

In many instances, however, considerable stress is placed on the couple's relationship because of the required periods of abstinence which are sometimes quite prolonged. This is particularly true in the case of women who have very irregular periods. Moreover, the various methods require considerable time for instruction and accurate records must often be kept. Also, it is difficult or impossible to determine the exact time of ovulation accurately if a woman has a vaginal or cervical infection. Any time the methods are not followed properly and consistently, failure rates tend to be rather high. Finally, it is obvious that unprotected intercourse will permit the transmission of STDs and HIV/AIDS.

8

Lactational Amenorrhea

MANY CENTURIES AGO, women discovered that they did not become pregnant again as long as they were breast-feeding their newborn babies. In earlier human societies, it was very important, for numerous reasons, for women to be able to plan their pregnancies. At that time, lactation was a major contributor to the spacing of children and it continues to be a significant form of birth control in many parts of the world today. Studies have found that lactational amenorrhea lasted for as long as two to three years in many countries. Of great interest are the hunter-gatherer nomadic !Kung women who practiced prolonged nursing. Anthropologists, using stopwatches, determined that these women's babies and toddlers nursed approximately two out of every fifteen minutes. Another pregnancy did not occur for about thirty-five months.

It has been estimated that in some parts of Africa and Asia breast-feeding has reduced the fertility rate on an average of 30 percent. Moreover, in certain cultures, it has been found that women who are lactating do not have sexual intercourse, and obviously the level of birth control effectiveness is extremely high in these areas.

Proper spacing of pregnancies is very important when looking at maternal and infant morbidity and mortality inasmuch as it is well known that repeated pregnancies at intervals of less than two years result in a higher incidence of preterm births, low-birth-weight babies, and infant deaths. Similarly, too frequent pregnancies produce a serious strain on a woman's health, particularly when they are superimposed on chronic malnutrition. Of course there are additional reasons, besides pregnancy prevention, for breast-feeding. It helps to establish better levels of mother-child bonding. There are also significant health benefits for babies who are fed on breast milk. It has been shown to provide not only excellent nutrition but also antibodies against certain infectious diseases and allergies. Finally, reports from areas where infant formulas have been aggressively promoted reveal that there is often a significant overdilution of the formula, often in the name of economy. Even worse, the formula is often diluted with contaminated water.

Effectiveness

The efficacy of lactational amenorrhea as a contraceptive method varies considerably. A number of factors that impact the duration and the effectiveness of breast-feeding have been identified. The most important of these is the frequency and the intensity of the suckling of the baby. Nursing, through a hormonal feedback to the central nervous system, stimulates and maintains the flow of breast milk. There is decreasing effectiveness when the baby begins to receive additional feedings such as infant formulas and foods. In this situation, the level of protection against pregnancy offered by lactation decreases because a woman is not fully lactating and ovulation tends to return more quickly. If the nutrition of the mother is poor, the impact of breast-feeding tends to continue longer.

The average effectiveness of lactational amenorrhea is about 90 percent, but only for those women who are fully breast-feeding. One study showed that if a woman was fully breast-feeding and had no resumption of menses, she would have a level of protection up to 98 percent for the first six months after delivery. However, it was noted that these high rates were obtainable only if a woman was exclusively breast-feeding at regular intervals including feeding during the night. Also this level of effectiveness occurred only if a woman did not begin to menstruate. Once menses returned, the possibility of ovulation and pregnancy went up sharply. In another study, it was estimated that a high level of effectiveness after six months required approximately fifteen or more nursing periods per day, each lasting ten minutes, and supplementation had to be limited to no more than 10 percent of the total food intake.

Studies have found that ovulation may sometimes occur in a lactating woman after three months and before she has her first menstrual period. Therefore, it is recommended that, in most instances, a contraceptive method be started at three months postpartum, even if a woman is fully breast-feeding. However, if a woman is not fully lactating but wishes to continue to breast-feed for the health benefits this will offer to her baby, she should use some form of birth control beginning the third postpartum week. Once a baby has been weaned, a woman's hormones gradually return to her previous prepregnancy pattern and ovulation will begin again approximately four weeks following the weaning of her baby.

Contraceptive Options

A woman can resume her use of any of the female barrier methods once postdelivery bleeding has stopped. Previously used caps and diaphragms should be checked to be sure that they still fit properly. Spermicides have an additional advantage; the vagina of a lactating woman can be drier than normal, and spermicides provide additional lubrication when intercourse is uncomfortable.

Male latex condoms are another good option for the lactating woman who wants pregnancy protection. When properly used, they can be quite effective; they are also her best defense against the transmission of STDs and HIV/AIDS.

IUDs can be inserted immediately after delivery or six to eight weeks later when the uterus has returned to its normal size. The currently available copper and progesterone devices are confined to the uterus; therefore they have no effect on lactation and are not a source of danger to the nursing infant. For reasons that are still unclear, women whose IUDs are put in while they are lactating experience fewer problems at the time of insertion and have lower rates of removals for pain and bleeding than are found in women whose IUDs are put in when they are not breast-feeding.

For many years oral contraceptives have been used during lactation. However, women who received the older high-dose pills often experienced a decrease in their breast milk. Even with the low-dose combination OCs, some decrease in the milk supply may occur. In general, if lactation is well established—and particularly if a woman has breast-fed successfully in the past—there is no significant adverse effect on either the amount or the content of the milk, and the nutrition and growth of the infants remain normal. Very small amounts of estrogen and progestin can be found in breast milk but in such tiny concentrations that they have no effect on the babies. A long-term Swedish study found no physical or mental abnormalities in children whose mothers had taken combination OCs while nursing.

At present, the minipill is most often advised for lactating women. In fact, this is the major reason today for the use of this form of hormonal contraception. While the progestin-only OCs are somewhat less effective in general than the combination products, in the presence of lactation, pregnancy prevention has been found to be highly successful. The progestin has been noted to increase the milk supply and to prolong the period of lactation and although found in small amounts in the breast milk, no damage to nursing infants has ever been documented.

The two most recently approved long-term progestin-only methods are also good contraceptive options. Subdermal implants have been used for a number of years in lactating women. In many countries they are inserted at the time of delivery; the FDA, however, recommends that they be used after lactation is well established, at about six weeks postpartum. DMPA has also been used in breast-feeding women for many years. Not only is it highly effective, but it usually prolongs lactation and increases the amount and protein content of breast milk. Neither of these methods has produced any adverse effects, either short- or long-term, on the babies of mothers using them.

If a woman is practicing periodic abstinence, she may encounter significant problems during the time she is lactating. This situation often requires special counseling. The typical markers of ovulation, particularly the changes in cervical mucus, are not present. This lack of verifiable evidence can lead to prolonged periods of abstinence.

A new problem related to breast-feeding has arisen, particularly in developing countries—the HIV/AIDS pandemic. Despite considerable research, it remains unclear as to how to assess the risk/benefit ratio of infant nutrition versus virus transmission. It is now well established that one-third of HIV-infected mothers pass the virus to their infants (vertical transmission) during pregnancy, delivery, or breast-feeding. The administration of antiviral agents during pregnancy and/or at delivery has been found to decrease the risk, but limitations of financial resources and adequate health-care delivery systems often make this option very difficult or impossible. In general, it is now recommended that breast-feeding be contraindicated only if adequate infant formula and clean water are readily available.

9

Additional Methods of Female Contraception

Vaginal Rings

FOR A NUMBER OF years, investigators have attempted to produce vaginal rings that would be useful as contraceptives. The ones that have been studied are made of silastic tubing, doughnut-shaped, about the size of a diaphragm. They contain either estrogen, estrogen and progestin, or progestin alone. They have been of two different types. One version contains a single core that allows a steady release of the hormones into the vagina. Another type has cores that contain individual layers of hormones designed to be released in sequence. Some are to be used for three weeks followed by removal for one week; others are good for several months of use. They do not need to be fitted and are inserted and removed by the woman herself.

Since 1972, the WHO has been testing a vaginal ring that releases 20 mcg of levonorgestrel a day for three months. It has a failure rate of about 4 percent; reasons for discontinuations have included menstrual problems, repeated expulsions, and vaginal irritation and discharge. Another progestin-only ring is being evaluated by the Population Council. It is a three-month device that releases about 10 mg of progesterone a day. It is being proposed for use by breast-feeding women.

A vaginal ring which will be manufactured with the name Nuva-Ring™ is now in the final stages of development. It measures 5.4 cm in diameter and 4.0 mm in thickness. It is made of ethylene vinylac-etate (EVA), which is soft and flexible, with estrogen and progestogen dispersed homogeneously inside the core of the ring. There is a daily release of 15 mcg of ethylene estradiol and 120 mcg of etonogestrel. Because it is in place constantly, the blood levels of the hormones remain stable.

The ring is inserted on the fifth day of a menstrual period. It is rec-ommended that condoms be used for the first seven days of the first cycle of ring use until adequate levels of the hormone have been released. The ring is inserted into the vagina but does not require any specified placement. It is left in for three weeks and then removed, following which withdrawal bleeding usually occurs in two or three days. One week later, the woman inserts a new ring.

The hormones from the ring are absorbed through the vagina and are picked up by the general circulation. They suppress ovulation and the progestin thickens the cervical mucus. Side effects are roughly comparable to those seen with OC use. One major difference is a low-ered incidence of nausea and vomiting because the hormones are absorbed through the vaginal walls and do not have to go through the upper gastrointestinal tract. The ring may be left in during sexual intercourse and very often neither partner is aware of its presence. However, if for some reason it becomes necessary to temporarily remove the ring, it should not be left out of the vagina for more than three hours. Most of the women in the studies using the ring reported that they liked the method.

Contraceptive Patches

Another fairly recent addition to the hormonal conceptive market is the contraceptive skin patch. This type of contraceptive usually con-tains both estrogen and a progestin. One of these patches, EVRA™, is seeking FDA approval. It is 20 cm^2 and it has been found to sup-press ovulation. The regimen consists of three patches, each lasting seven days. After three weeks the woman goes without the patch for one week. Withdrawal bleeding usually occurs during this time, and then the woman begins the next cycle of patches. Preliminary studies show that, in general, compliance with the patch is better than with daily oral administration. It is believed that this approach will result in higher levels of acceptability and effectiveness.

Contraceptive Gels

Another transdermal method that is being studied is the contraceptive gel. This approach has been tried with a number of different steroids, which are mixed with the gel and then applied to the skin. In 1992 it was reported that a progestin—ST-1435—administered in a gel was released at a rate of 0.8 mg per day, which effectively suppressed ovulation.

Female Sterilization

In 1978, male and female sterilizations moved ahead of the pill for the first time as the number one method of family planning both in the United States and worldwide; sterilization maintains that position in many areas even today. It has been estimated that approximately one-quarter of American women are protected against unwanted pregnancy by sterilization procedures; 18 percent of these are female procedures and 8 percent are male. The incidence of female sterilization increases with age. About 33 percent of women age thirty to thirty-four, 45 percent of women age thirty-five to thirty-nine, and 51 percent of women age forty to forty-four have had a tubal ligation. Close to 700,000 American women request this form of permanent contraception each year.

Sterilization procedures in the female are more difficult to perform than sterilization procedures in the male. In order to reach the fallopian tubes, the surgeon must access the abdominal cavity either through the abdominal wall or through the vagina. Although sterilizations can be carried out at any time, the majority of the procedures are done immediately after the delivery of a baby, often under the same general anesthetic. This has been the time of choice for several reasons. First, the fallopian tubes are high in the abdomen as a result of the pregnancy; therefore they can easily be reached by making a small incision or using a laparoscope. Since the woman is usually already in a health-care facility, the sterilization adds little time to her hospital stay, and she does not have to return at a later probably less convenient date to have the procedure.

With the advent of new medical technology, particularly the fiber optics such as the laparoscope and culdoscope, the sterilizing procedures are increasingly easy to perform. Use of these instruments dramatically reduces the time required to do a traditional laparotomy (the surgical opening of the abdomen) and is less extensive and safer. They have made it easier to do tubal ligations at any point in time, and sterilizations are often performed in outpatient facilities, frequently under local anesthesia.

Numerous surgical approaches to sterilization have been developed over the years. The most commonly used procedure has been the Pomeroy method. A loop of the tube is brought up and tied off, and the loop is then removed. A number of other procedures including the Irving, Madlener, Aldridge, and Uchida methods—named after their inventors—have been used. They all involve blockage of the tubes, either by surgical division or burying of the tubes under the lining tissues of the abdomen. A somewhat different approach is the Kroener method. This consists of removing the fimbriated (outer) end of the tube and then tying off the stump. Finally, one technique, less commonly practiced today, is the cornual resection; the tube is cut and tied off at the cornua—the place where it enters the uterus.

With the development of laparoscopy, a number of techniques were developed and are now widely employed. These include tubal electrocautery, unipolar diathermy, bipolar diathermy, thermal coagulation, and tubal obstruction methods using a variety of rings and clips. In addition, several procedures performed through the vagina have been used. While they do not require an abdominal surgical procedure, they have a higher rate of pelvic infection.

Researchers have for many years attempted to perfect a procedure involving the application of chemicals either into the uterine cavity or into the tubes to produce scar tissue causing an obstruction.

They have used multiple agents. Quinacrine has been the most commonly employed, and it is currently undergoing a number of clinical trials. Other chemicals that have been tried in the past include phenol and methylcyanoacrylate. So far none of the procedures has been both simple to perform and consistently highly effective. There have also been attempts to place devices into the tubes, installing them through the uterine cavity; however, many of these devices did not stay in place and they were only moderately successful. Despite this, attempts to design tubal plugs continue.

Morbidity and mortality rates are very low with the currently used forms of female sterilization. A review published in 1989 covering nine hundred thousand procedures found only three deaths. In 1992, data from a study carried out in fifty countries reported a mortality rate of 3.7 per 100,000 procedures. Most of the deaths were related to the complications of anesthesia, not the procedure itself. A second, less-common cause was a postoperative infection, including cases of tetanus. This was most common in procedures that were carried out in developing countries under less than ideal surgical conditions.

Pregnancy rates following sterilization procedures have classically been reported as less than 1 percent. Women have been told that their chances for pregnancy after their surgery were minimal to absent. However, this assumption has recently been challenged. A study carried out in the United States by the CDC has assessed the effectiveness and risks of a number of forms of sterilization over a ten-year period of time. In this study, called the Collaborative Review of Sterilization (CREST), 10,685 women were followed for up to fourteen years. Their procedures were performed between the years of 1978 and 1986 at sixteen major medical centers in nine cities. As a result of this monumental work, extensive data are now available on the efficacy and side effects of each of the various methods that were evaluated. The overall figure obtained for cumulative failure was 1.9 percent, nearly twice the number as was traditionally believed.

The implications of these data have been considerable in that it is no longer possible to tell women that they are virtually 100 percent safe after their sterilization procedure has been done. It is also now recognized that failures may occur as late as 10 to 15 years after the procedure. This is not common; however, it does occur and women need to be aware of the potential. This new information has, to some degree, increased the use of highly effective long-term but reversible methods of contraception such as IUDs, implants, and injections. Women now more often see them as viable alternatives.

The CREST data showed that failure rates were related to age; younger women have the highest rates and the rates get progressively lower in women approaching menopause. The study found that the highest incidence of regret and of requests for reversals occurred in the younger age group. Other data coming out of the CREST study showed that the incidence of ectopic pregnancies following sterilizations varied by the type of procedure that was performed; it was most common after the bipolar method. In fact, ectopic pregnancies constituted one-third of the total failures and the frequency increased progressively over the ten-year period of observation. Therefore it is important that women know of this possibility. They should understand the signs and symptoms of ectopic pregnancy so that they can seek immediate medical care in case any of them should develop.

The possible existence of something known as the post-tubal syndrome has been debated for many years and was also analyzed for in the CREST study. Several earlier studies had found that there were increased episodes of abnormal bleeding after sterilization procedures, both at the time of the menstrual periods and between periods. The CREST data have shown that there is no bleeding pattern of this type, regardless of the method that was used. One probable reason for the earlier misperception was the fact that many women had been using the OCs up to the time of their surgery. In all probability, the change from normal to abnormal cycles was due to stopping the use of the oral contraceptives, not to the sterilization procedure itself.

Several years after surgery, in one study, about 10 percent of the women expressed feelings of regret about their loss of fertility. This was particularly true of younger women and those who had their procedures done after a delivery, especially after cesarean sections. However, only 0.2 percent of these women actually asked to have a surgical reversal. The number of requests for reversal also varied by the age of the woman; those under thirty years were twice as likely to ask to have their fertility restored as those who were older. Also women who had had a change in their marital status were found to consider sterilization reversal three times more often than women whose marital status remained unchanged.

The possibility of reversing a sterilization procedure varies by the type of surgery that was performed. For women whose tubes have had minimal damage, success in reversal procedures can be quite high—up to 70 percent. On the other hand, if large portions of the tubes have been destroyed, the chances of a successful reversal are much smaller. In addition, approximately 5 percent of the women who have had reversal procedures performed have subsequently developed ectopic pregnancies.

A common theory from the past was that having a tubal sterilization would increase the chances that a woman would need to have a hysterectomy at some time in the future, possibly due to interference with the blood supply to the ovaries or to the uterus. However, data from the CREST study indicated that when compared to the rate found in nonsterilized women there was no increase in the frequency of hysterectomy after sterilization. The current theory is that the hysterectomies that were performed in the group that had been sterilized were related to the aging of the women and the consequently higher incidence of various types of age-related gynecological disorders.

Still another question, raised in previous years by several small studies, has been whether or not tubal sterilizations are related to the subsequent development of cancer of the uterus, ovaries, and breasts. However, more recent studies have shown no association between these procedures and the development of either breast or endometrial cancer. In fact, in the case of the ovary, there are now data suggesting that the risk of developing cancer of the ovary may actually be decreased following tubal ligation. Additional research is being carried out to see if, first, this is true, and second, if so, why.

Douching

For centuries women have attempted to wash the ejaculate out of their vaginas using a wide variety of different and sometimes dangerous products as douching materials. (Coca-Cola was a very popular choice, particularly among teenagers, several years ago.) These attempts have usually been highly unsuccessful. Until recently, the reason for the high failure rates was not clear. However, with more detailed investigations of the female reproductive tract immediately following sexual intercourse, it has now been shown that sperm can be found in the fallopian tubes within ninety seconds after ejaculation. Clearly, even Olympic sprinters would have considerable difficulty getting to a douche bag or other douching material within that time frame.

Moreover, douching has been suspected for a number of years to be a cause of infection and PID, possibly resulting in scarring of the tubes and leading to ectopic pregnancies. Therefore, as it is both ineffective and possibly dangerous, douching should be discouraged as a contraceptive method.

Female Immunologic Methods

Many years and dollars have been spent looking at whether it would be possible to immunize women against some part of the reproductive process and cause them to be temporarily unable to conceive. A number of vaccines have been tried, the one receiving the most attention being against human chorionic gonadotropin (hCG), a hormone that is necessary to maintain a pregnancy. Another approach has been to develop antibodies against part of the egg, the early embryo, or sperm. However, there are many concerns about the use of agents of this type because it has never been determined what impact any of them might have on other body tissues. To be generally useful, a vaccine would have to be not only safe and effective, but also reversible. While extensive research has been carried out, there remains considerable doubt that a contraceptive vaccine will become practical and available in the near future.

10

Male Contraception

It was reported in the *Guinness Book of World Records* that the most prolific man in history was Ismail the Bloodthirsty, who was the Sharifian Emperor of Morocco from 1672 to 1727. He claimed to have fathered 888 children with the help of some 500 young women in his harem. Present-day scientists have calculated that to do this, he would have to have had sexual relations with 4.8 women every day for forty years, and have a constant supply of millions of viable sperm—no small feat!

Ever since the invention of the microscope, scientists have conducted thousands of studies in the attempt to learn more about basic reproductive structures and functions. Among this group were animal and human semen. Some early researchers provided interesting, somewhat fanciful, descriptions of sperm. They were variously reported as being donkey-shaped and as looking like miniature men. Eventually, they were accurately described, but then new questions arose.

First, scientists had to determine how many sperm had to be present in an ejaculate in order to produce a pregnancy, given that only a single sperm would ultimately be allowed to enter an egg. Normal values for many years ranged from twenty million to one hundred million sperm/ml. For a time, researchers believed that any count lower than ten million indicated infertility. More recently, however, it was found that in some cases even fewer than one million could produce fertilization. This fact once was documented by obtaining sperm counts of men waiting in obstetrical units for their wives to deliver—clearly accepting a basic underlying assumption.

Eventually scientists realized that the number of sperm was not the sole criterion for determining fertility. Equally important was their structure (normal or misshapen), motility (ability to swim), and viability (alive or dead) as well as the composition and volume of the ejaculate. A measurement of fertility commonly used today is the motile sperm count—the number of sperm times the percent motility.

Basic information drawn from hundreds of studies has provided a much improved understanding of male reproductive function. It has also led to attempts to find safe and effective ways in which to control male fertility.

Withdrawal

Withdrawal (coitus interruptus) is commonly thought to be the earliest widely used method of contraception. It is also thought to have been primarily responsible for the avoidance of pregnancy in the nineteenth century, prior to the development of our modern forms of birth control. To practice withdrawal, when a man realizes that he is close to orgasm, he removes his penis from the vagina and allows ejaculation to occur outside. This method is still frequently and widely used. However, it is unacceptable to some men for both emotional reasons and for the relatively lower levels of effectiveness, being roughly the same as the barrier contraceptives. Only about half of the men who attempt to use this technique are consistently able to control the timing of their ejaculations; and, clearly, it is totally unsuitable for men with premature or early ejaculation.

The earliest written reference to withdrawal, noted in chapter 1 of this volume, was the time that Onan was told by his father, Judah, to have intercourse with the wife of his dead brother, "to raise up seed" for him. However, Onan refused to do so, and "spilled his seed on the ground." There are still theological arguments about why this was a sin—lack of family duty, disobedience, or greed. In any event, it led to the only known mortality from the use of withdrawal since it "did displease Yahweh, who killed him."

The prophet Mohammed pointed out that "had this practice been injurious, it would have harmed the Romans and Persians." He felt that withdrawal was acceptable, however, only if a woman agreed to its use. In the Koran, coitus interruptus was found to be acceptable but, in the Jewish community, there was a belief that withdrawal constituted killing of a life in miniature form. Islam gave withdrawal the name of *azl* and found it acceptable. In 1270, the bishop of Lyons said "the sin against nature occurs when one contrives or consents that the seed be spilled in a place other than that allotted by nature."

Over the years some very picturesque phrases have been coined to describe withdrawal. The Talmud calls it "threshing inside and winnowing outside" and in East Yorkshire, England, it is described as "going to Beverley and getting off at Cottingham."

There have also been many myths about the physical and mental effects of withdrawal. For many years, the practice of coitus interruptus has elicited comments, both positive and negative, from numerous members of the medical and religious communities. At one time, it was felt that men using coitus interruptus as a contraceptive technique would become impotent; some urologists were sure that these men would develop prostate disease. In 1878, a lecturer at the British Medical Association concluded that moral and physical evils would follow the use of what he called "conjugal onanism." He claimed that it caused numerous disorders including leukorrhea, metritis, sterility, nymphomania, galloping cancer, and suicide. Many of the side effects that were blamed on the use of withdrawal were most likely not a problem with the method itself, but rather the result of religious condemnation, which made the practice unacceptable.

Clearly, this form of birth control was widely known and widely practiced for many centuries. The only methods available to couples to control their fertility during the eighteenth century were abstinence, abortion, and withdrawal. Historic demographers have looked into the practice of withdrawal and have documented its impact over the years throughout the world. Multiple studies have been carried out in England, Scandinavia, and France. The primary method of assessment has been reviews of records of births, baptisms, marriages, and deaths; the effectiveness of withdrawal has been very evident in these records. For example, it was noted that in nineteenth-century Spain birth rates were 30 percent lower than those in Russia at the same time. Researchers believe that these differences reflect the widespread use of withdrawal in Spain. Actually the decline in births noted in a number of countries occurred before any of our semimodern methods of birth control became available. In fact, even when some of the earlier contraceptive techniques such as condoms, caps, and spermicides were developed, they most likely played a relatively minor role compared to withdrawal until the twentieth century.

Numerous studies have been carried out in various parts of the world looking at birth rates in terms of social class, size of community, religious backgrounds, and a number of other socio-demographic factors. In 1949, the Royal Commission on Population in Britain did a survey to investigate contraceptive usage patterns and results. They reported that no significant difference had been found in family size between individuals using appliances and nonappliance methods; withdrawal was clearly the most important of the nonappliance techniques. Another study, this one done in Princeton, found a failure rate of 17 percent for coitus interruptus as compared with 14 percent for the condom and diaphragm, and 38 percent for periodic abstinence. Still another survey, this one from Indianapolis, showed a failure rate of only 10 percent, all other methods available at that time averaging 12 percent.

More recently, there has been renewed interest in the evaluation of withdrawal as a contraceptive method, resulting in a clearer pattern of the role that it has played over the years. For example, in the 1970s, the World Fertility Survey (WFS) carried out a detailed study and came up with some very interesting data, which it presented at the United Nations Fund for Population Activity (UNFPA)/WHO meeting in London in 1983. It found a high percentage of the use of withdrawal in many countries—60 percent in Jamaica and 67 percent in Hungary. The survey found greater use of coitus interruptus in developed countries than in developing countries, but in both it was clearly an important method.

In 1931, Dr. Abraham Stone suggested that the use of coitus interruptus could not be a very effective form of contraception inasmuch as sperm were present in the preejaculate. To test this hypothesis, he collected preejaculate fluid from a number of men, and, indeed, sperm were there; however, they were very few in number, only occasional specimens having more than a few sperm. We now know from current research that it is probably impossible for fertilization to occur in this situation; these fluids contain very small numbers of sperm and a very large number (millions) of sperm have to be deposited in the vagina to produce a pregnancy.

Another observation suggesting that the sperm in preejaculatory fluid probably have a very low order of effectiveness is the fact that these particular sperm have been present within the man's reproductive tract at body temperature since the last ejaculation. Normal body temperatures are well known to interfere with the ability of sperm to fertilize an egg, as noted in men with undescended testicles, since temperatures in the scrotum are considerably lower than in the abdomen. (Two additional forms of birth control have been suggested based on this information. The first is the use of the jock strap, a device which holds the scrotum up against the warmer lower abdomen. The second is prolonged sitting in hot bath water. While interesting in concept, neither one has been subjected to serious scientific scrutiny.)

According to estimates from multiple studies, withdrawal has been used by more couples and has averted more pregnancies than a number of the more current methods, including condoms, vaginal barriers, injectables, and implants. It is now well established that coitus interruptus was the major reason for the declines in fertility that occurred during the period of industrialization in the West, the economic depression in the 1930s in Europe, and after World War II in Eastern Europe. Each of these represents a modern society that was among the first to achieve zero population growth.

Condoms

Men have used condoms for many years. The original condoms, several centuries ago, were made out of a number of plant and animal materials. They have been associated in the past with a very negative image, being used primarily for venereal disease (VD) prevention. They were often associated with prostitution and extramarital sex. Today the condom's image has become a bit more positive. Like other barrier contraceptives, condoms are increasingly being used not only for the prevention of pregnancy, but also, and even more often, because of concerns over the rising rates of STDs, particularly HIV/AIDS. In fact, in some areas of the world, they are the method of choice. It has been estimated that more than 6 billion condoms were distributed in 1990, far fewer than the number calculated to be needed to prevent unwanted pregnancies and STDs. A distribution goal of more than 20 billion has been set for the millennium by some public health associations.

Description

There are several types of condoms. The most commonly used ones are made out of latex rubber with either a plain or reservoir tip. Natural animal membrane or "skin" condoms, made from the intestines of sheep, have been used in the past. Many men preferred them because they interfered less with sensation. Also they could be cleaned and used more than one time. However, it has been found that the smaller viruses such as HIV and hepatitis B can pass through the walls of these condoms; therefore, they are no longer being recommended. Some condoms are manufactured with additives such as spermicides and lubricants. Others are made in bright colors, are decorated, or have ribbing to increase stimulation during use.

A number of studies have been carried out looking for ways to improve condoms. One of the materials used in these trials was polyurethane. There were several reasons for this selection. Allergies to latex have proved to be more common than was previously thought, and, on occasion, they can be dangerous and even fatal. For example, one study in a group of hospital employees found an 8 to 17 percent incidence of latex-induced asthma. Polyurethane is stronger than latex. It was thought to be possibly more user-friendly since it is transparent, odorless, and thinner and more resistant to the adverse effects of some lubricants.

In 1999, the results of the first randomized controlled clinical trial comparing the effectiveness and acceptability of latex and polyurethane condoms were published. The study found that latex and polyurethane failure rates were 6.3 percent and 4.8 percent, respectively—essentially the same. From the point of view of acceptability, the clinical trial did not find polyurethane condoms to be an improvement over latex; in fact, they had a number of less desirable attributes. Breakage rates were ten times higher with polyurethane (4 percent versus 0.4 percent) and slippage rates were four times higher (4.5 percent versus 1.2 percent). Moreover, discontinuation rates were two-thirds higher for the polyurethane condoms—not only because of breakage and slippage problems but also because men found them less attractive and harder to put on. However, users also reported that they caused less local irritation, had a more pleasant odor, and allowed better sensitivity than the latex condoms.

Many laboratory tests have been developed to test the strength of condoms under different pressures and conditions. They are blown up to determine the pressure it takes to make them burst. Permeability testing of condoms, both the older latex and newer polyurethane, is also being carried out, assessing their potential ability to block the transmission of HIV and other STDs. One such study, using dyes and gases such as helium and nitrogen, found that polyurethane film was less permeable than latex. This study concluded that because dyes and gases are blocked by polyurethane, it is unlikely that the larger STD organisms could get through.

Usage

It is important to apply a condom before there is any contact with the vulva or penetration of the vagina. Condoms should be unrolled to their full length, leaving a half inch free at the tip unless the type with a reservoir tip is being used. Contraceptive jellies and creams may be used as lubricants and for additional contraceptive protection. Following ejaculation, it is important to remove the penis from the vagina while it is still erect, holding carefully to the rim of the condom, so that there will be no spillage of semen. It should be checked after removal for breakage and then discarded.

In July 2001, NIH issued a report of a study on condoms that it cosponsored with the FDA and AID. A group of twenty-eight experts ananlyzed 138 peer-reviewed studies; they concluded that correct and consistent use of male latex condoms helped to prevent the transmission of HIV/AIDS in both men and women, of gonorrhea in men, and also offered good protection against pregnancy. The data on other STDs were insufficient to draw valid conclusions.

Other recent studies have demonstrated a reduction in the risk of transmission of genital herpes, gonorrhea, and chlamydia to women with condom use. They also have reported a lower risk of transmissin of gonorrhea and chlamydia to men.

Although condoms are, at the moment, the best protection against STD transmission other than abstinence, studies unfortunately show that both men and women who are at high risk for STDs do not necessarily move to the use of condoms as quickly as their circumstances would suggest. Some of the most vulnerable people in today's society are not protecting themselves by the use of condoms.

Advantages and Disadvantages

Condom use is increasing because of growing concern about the rapidly rising rates of STDs. Condoms are available over-the-counter and they are easy to use and dispose of. Men who wish to assume their share of the responsibility for preventing pregnancy and STD transmission often elect to use condoms. Men who have premature ejaculations also find condoms useful to prolong the duration of sexual intercourse. There are no serious side effects from the use of the condom. Occasional sensitivity is found to the latex rubber, the lubricant, or the spermicide.

Condoms have the disadvantage of having to be used with each act of intercourse. Many men complain about the need to put the condom on following erection; others say that they interfere with pleasurable sensations.

Effectiveness

The best effectiveness rates of condoms used without spermicides is reported to be as high as 98 percent, the average effectiveness being about 88 percent. Effectiveness rates depend on proper use and are increased by the addition of a female barrier method. A 1999 study of serodiscordant couples (one partner with HIV and the other uninfected) showed that condoms are equally effective in the prevention of HIV transmission and pregnancy. It was previously believed that condom failures were due, in almost all instances, to incorrect usage. Newer evidence, however, suggests that breakage and slippage rates are actually higher than had previously been thought.

Male Sterilization

A vasectomy is performed in the male to render him permanently incapable of producing a pregnancy. Vasectomies are carried out less often than are female-sterilizing procedures. However, in the male, the surgery is much safer, simpler, and less expensive. Both male and female sterilization procedures are very safe and very effective. However, the costs are quite different, the average cost of a vasectomy being $500 as compared with $2,500 for a female tubal ligation.

Male sterilizations are performed on the vas deferens, the tubes that carry sperm from the testes to the penis. A number of different ways have been devised to block the vas. Surgical procedures are usually done under local anesthesia in an office or outpatient facility. The man may go home immediately and actually goes back to normal activities within a few days. It is important that men having a vasectomy be warned that they are not immediately sterile. Sperm that have already been produced will stay in the reproductive tract for about six weeks. Couples are advised to use another form of birth control for either twelve weeks or until the man has had approximately twenty ejaculations. It is usually wise to have a check of the semen several weeks after a procedure has been performed to make sure that the operation has been successful and that there are no sperm present in the semen.

In general, vasectomies should be considered to be permanent. Attempts have been made to reverse the procedures and restore fertility; however, these are usually quite expensive, involve considerable surgery, and have not been notably successful. Reversal should be done within the first ten years after the original operation. Studies have shown that in the event of a reversal, even though sperm may again be found in the ejaculate, the potential for producing a pregnancy, for some reason, perhaps due to some autoimmune response, remains limited.

Techniques allowing reversibility have been sought for many years on the assumption that it would increase the use of the procedure. The most common approach has been to put a small device in the vas, removing it when fertility was again desired. These have included such things as suture material, silicone threads, plugs, and beads. One interesting device made of gold had a valve that was supposed to be turned off and on through the scrotum; it turned out not to be very effective.

A more practical device is the Shug. It consists of two hollow silicone plugs held together by a nylon suture and blocked at both ends. The plugs are either 0.7 mm or 1 mm in length; they fit snugly in the vas without exerting a lot of pressure. The suture is left outside the vas and used for removal. Other techniques have included clips put on the vas, one of which released copper. The plan was to remove them if and when the subject decided he wanted the return of his fertility. The major problems with most of the devices put inside the vas were twofold. First, they were not sufficiently effective, because the vas would dilate around them, and, second, they often were not reversible because scarring caused by the foreign body produced permanent blockage. Additional studies have been done using metals, chemicals, heat, and electro-coagulation in attempts to produce scarring and closure of the vas. None of these alternative methods has proved to be highly successful and therefore none has been widely used.

The traditional vasectomy procedures are carried out by making an incision over each vas deferens, grasping them and tying them off after a section has been removed. (Some surgeons prefer to use a single incision.) Many attempts have been made to make vasectomies easier. One approach is the "no-scalpel" technique, a procedure invented in China in 1974. It has the advantage of requiring only a small puncture over the vas instead of a surgical incision; special instruments have been designed for this type of procedure. It is less traumatic, there is less pain and swelling, and the recovery time is very short. About 30 percent of the vasectomies done in the United States are now carried out using this method.

Complications at the time of surgery and immediately after the sterilization procedures are usually minor. The most common of these are pain, bruising, and swelling of the scrotum. On occasion, there may be bleeding resulting in a hematoma (a collection of blood) in the scrotum. Rarely, an infection may occur in some part of the male genital tract. An inflammation resulting from sperm leaking into the surrounding tissue known as a sperm granuloma may develop.

The use of vasectomy has been limited, particularly in certain cultures, because of a number of fears. Predominant among these are the concerns that some men have that the procedure will make them more feminine, will cause the pitch of their voices to go up, will decrease their interest in sex, and will interfere with their ability to have erections and ejaculations. Increased anxiety also stems from the fact that in some languages the word for *sterilization* is the same as the word for *castration*. One interesting approach, found to be very useful with illiterate men, is to liken the procedure to removing all of the fish from a river: the water continues to flow unchanged, but the fish are gone.

In the past it has also been suggested that a vasectomy might increase a man's risk of autoimmune diseases, testicular and prostate cancer, or heart disease. However, multiple studies by the WHO and the U.S. National Institutes of Health (NIH) have not borne out these risks. In fact, statistics show that vasectomy is a very safe operation. In the United States, no deaths have ever been reported from male sterilization procedures. However, deaths have been reported in other areas of the world when these procedures were done under far less than adequate medical conditions; these deaths usually result from infections, including tetanus. A study looking at possible cardiovascular risks was carried out among U.S. physicians who had had vasectomies. The data showed no increase in myocardial infarction, angina, or stroke, even fifteen years after the procedure.

Medical Approaches

Considerable time, money, and effort have gone into the search for safe and effective forms of contraception for men. To date no single product has been found that is entirely satisfactory. Contraception in the male is a very different proposition than contraception in the female. Whereas women produce only one egg a month, men constantly turn out sperm by the millions. The goal in men, yet to be realized, is to find products that will produce infertility without affecting libido and potency. To be totally protective, a male birth control method must reach two goals. First, a man's sperm count must go down to zero; second, it must *remain* at zero. A number of agents that were studied appeared to be successful for a period of time, but then the "escape phenomenon" occurred: sperm again began to be present in the ejaculate. This happened without any perceptible change being noted or any change in the products being used. Needless to say, it was impossible to document this in any easy way and the diagnosis was usually made by finding a pregnancy.

Many years ago, a product that appeared to meet both of the goals was developed and tested in a prison population. However, once the chemical was tested in the general population, it was found to behave like Antabuse (disulfiram)—a drug developed to treat alcoholism—both drugs induced severe symptoms including nausea and vomiting whenever any form of alcohol was ingested. Further study of this drug as a contraceptive was not pursued.

Numerous studies have looked into the effects of various hormones in the male. Although sperm counts were found to decrease with the use of estrogen, the results of treatment were not predictable or constant. Even more disturbing, many of the subjects began to note feminizing changes in their appearances. They started to grow breasts, feminine curves, and a higher vocal register. They also had a considerable loss of libido and frequently were unable to develop erections and to have ejaculations. Even more ominous was the finding that men being given estrogen for the treatment of prostate cancer had an increased risk of myocardial infarction. Needless to say, this approach to male contraception was also short-lived.

A number of hormones have been looked at as possible male contraceptives including testosterone, the primary sexual hormone in men, either used alone or with other hormones. However, testosterone cannot be given by mouth since it is immediately broken down by the liver. Therefore studies were carried out by the WHO and NIH for more than a decade, giving testosterone at weekly intervals by injection; the use of testosterone pellets and microcapsules was also explored. One study was carried out using pellets placed under the skin of the abdomen and replaced every twelve weeks. It was found that azoospermia (no sperm in the ejaculate) was not always achieved and it could take a number of weeks of treatment before the sperm count began to go down. Also some men noted acne, weight gain, and mood changes.

One of the most promising approaches has been the use of a combination of progestins to block the pituitary hormones (which stimulate the development of sperm), and androgen (to maintain sexuality). One such study looked at data gathered from sixty-six men treated with a progestin, desogestrel, and a pellet of testosterone. Nine of the subjects dropped out before the twenty-four week study was over complaining of symptoms such as headache, acne, increased appetite, and weight gain. However, others in the study liked this particular form of contraception and asked to continue it.

In China in the 1960s it was noted that farmers who had been exposed to cottonseed oil became ill and also infertile. This led to a clinical trial of gossypol, a nonsteroidal compound found in cottonseeds, as a male contraceptive in China in 1972; it was reported to be effective but to have a considerable number of adverse side effects. These included dangerously low levels of blood potassium, nausea and vomiting, fatigue, and possible adverse effects on the liver and heart. Gossypol acts directly on the developing sperm, and the impact of the drug may persist after stopping treatment; approximately 25 percent of the men who used this product over a long period of time failed to regain their fertility.

Given the wide-ranging toxicity found in many animal studies coupled with the problems found in human research, further investigation of the original product was not warranted. However, evaluations of drugs related to gossypol are underway to look at these drugs' effectiveness, reversibility, and, particularly, toxicity. It remains to be seen if any of these will turn out to be promising in the future.

In general, it appears that men are increasingly willing to accept personal responsibility for birth control, as witnessed by the growing number of vasectomies. There has also been a significantly greater use of condoms, although the percentage of condom use related to contraception as compared to STD prevention is unknown.

If and when an excellent male contraceptive is developed, several key questions will remain. The issue of the possible acceptance of a contraceptive pill was addressed by a study of 155 men in California; it was found that 56 percent said that they would use one, 19 percent said they might, 18 percent said probably not, and 7 percent said absolutely not.

Another interesting aspect to male contraception is the question, would women be willing to entrust their protection against unwanted pregnancy entirely to their partner(s)? Even if highly safe and effective methods could be found, surveys have suggested that they would not be universally accepted to the exclusion of female contraceptives.

Male Immunological Methods

Scientists have long searched for methods to develop antibodies against some component of sperm. Certain antibodies have been developed that are apparently successful in primates; their fertility was considerably reduced and was restored when the injections were discontinued. However, studies looking at the possibility of producing the same desired effect in the human male are very complex and have not been carried out. It appears highly unlikely that an agent of this type will be developed and made available any time in the near future.

Male Reactions

A number of different surveys have evaluated reactions of men to women's use of oral contraceptives. The responses were quite varied, depending primarily on the basic psychodynamics of the particular individuals. Many husbands or partners were happy that the fear of pregnancy had been removed, and several studies reported that the frequency of sexual intercourse went up when women started OC use. Also, a couple's emotional attitudes toward each other often improved. In addition, men who had been using condoms were frequently relieved not to have to continue to use a coitally related method they did not like.

On the other hand, not all the men studied responded favorably to the institution of effective female contraception. Some felt threatened by the fact that a woman now had control over her fertility; some men resented the independence of behavior that reliable methods of birth control could give their female partners. Other men who were emotionally and sexually insecure developed major psychological problems when their wives or sexual partners began to take the pill; previously the establishment of a pregnancy had provided these men with proof of their virility and fertility.

Numerous reports were published in the medial literature and in the lay press about the effects of the use of the OCs on men who had made a very poor psychosexual adjustment. Released from the fear of pregnancy, many women became much more sexually aggressive. In most instances this was appreciated but in a few cases it posed a major threat to a man whose sexuality was already borderline. In fact, there were a number of cases reported of men who actually became impotent when their wives began taking OCs. Some extremely insecure men became very apprehensive, almost to the point of paranoia, at the thought that their wives were now free from the risk of unwanted pregnancy and, therefore, might be more likely to have sexual intercourse with other men. Some of these individuals were reported to have become physically violent toward their wives as a direct consequence of these overwhelming fears.

Thus, it was found that the removal of the fear of pregnancy, while basically advantageous, could also mobilize fears and conflicts in basic sexuality on the part of either the male or the female or, in some instances, both. However, these extreme reactions were found to occur primarily in individuals who had already exhibited neurotic behavior patterns prior to the initiation of contraception, and effective birth control methods were often made the scapegoat for preexisting long-term interpersonal problems.

11

The Current Status of Contraception

The Need for Better Contraception

Surveys on contraceptive usage show that existing methods are failing to meet the needs of many Americans as well as those living in other parts of the world. To meet their reproductive needs, people require different types of contraceptives at different stages of their lives. Statistics show that current techniques are either inappropriate or inadequate for the attitudes, behavior, and lifestyles of many individuals. Regardless of a method's effectiveness, if it is not utilized because of medical, personal, or social reasons, it will have little impact.

Additional evidence of our failure to provide good contraceptive care is the fact that induced abortion is one of the most common surgical procedures performed—not only in the United States but also around the world. Studies have shown that about one-quarter of the pregnancies in the United States are terminated by elective abortions, amounting to more than 1.3 million each year. Moreover, it has been estimated that 43 percent of American women will have at least one induced abortion by the age of forty-five.

In an earlier era, parents could not assume that even half of their children would live to the age of maturity, a situation which unfortunately still exists in many areas of the developing world. Because the children were needed to help with the family chores and to support their parents' old age, it was necessary to have a large number of offspring to ensure that enough of them would survive. This was particularly true in those cultures in which it was absolutely essential to have at least one living son. (With improved medical care and higher infant survival rates, the current trend is clearly toward smaller families in many, if not most, countries.)

Not only do other new safe and effective technologies have to be developed, but also another equally important factor in the acceptance and continued utilization of contraception is the quality of our medical care and delivery systems. The unmet need, particularly in some developing countries, is enormous. Millions of women who would use birth control measures if they were available are unable to do so. The training and attitudes of health-care providers, the amount and type of education provided to the public, and the attitudes of couples toward sexuality, childbearing, and contraception all play key roles in how well birth control measures are utilized.

Another clear indication of the current rather poor contraceptive situation in the United States is the estimate that approximately 3 million unplanned pregnancies occur each year, about 2 million of them the result of contraceptive failure. About half of the 1 million-plus abortions done each year stem from the same cause. Taking abortion data into account, the failure rates of our currently available methods are probably even higher than those that are usually cited. While unintended pregnancies occur in women of all ages, the highest rates are among teenagers and women over forty. These groups also have the highest abortion rates, as would have been predicted.

Another well-recognized outcome of the lack of appropriate or acceptable contraceptives has been the rising rates of sterilization. Often, when a couple has achieved their desired family size, they still have twenty or more years of potential fertility ahead of them. As a result, they are increasingly moving toward either male or female sterilization procedures that are often permanent, despite new and better methods of reversal.

Unfortunately, it is not widely appreciated that contraceptive use can lead not only to the prevention of unwanted pregnancy, but also to a lowered need for abortion and a reduction in the transmission of

STDs. Some contraceptive methods can prevent a significant number of medical conditions and malignancies as well the numerous health risks—for both mothers and their babies—associated with too many pregnancies and too frequent childbearing.

There are many socioeconomic factors that support the need for safe, effective contraceptives. For example, if a country can slow its population growth, it can then speed up its social and economic development. Rapid population growth is increasingly recognized as the most important contributor to the depletion of our natural resources, to our escalating environmental pollution, and to multiple forms of social stress. Clearly, inadequate attention has been given to the global benefits that might be derived from increased contraceptive usage. In fact, active opposition to all forms of fertility regulation continues with an utter disregard for the huge price that will have to be paid by future generations. Unfortunately, evaluations of current contraceptive products focus primarily on safety, efficacy, and the risk/benefit ratio as applied only to individuals, without adequate regard for their potential global impact.

Finally, the introduction of any new method has been documented to increase overall contraceptive use. Thus, there is an incremental advantage to finding and introducing additional safe, effective, and acceptable forms of family planning.

The Current Status of Contraceptive Research and Development

It is clear that there is a problem with regard to the development of new contraceptive techniques in the United States. While some new products have been developed, they are basically very similar to those previously approved; they represent only relatively minor improvements in terms of safety, effectiveness, and acceptability and are often referred to as "me-too" products. The congressional Office of Technology Assessment (OTA) recognized and evaluated this deficit in a 1980 survey. Its report, published in 1981, concluded that nine new methods would probably be available before 1990. In point of fact, only three of these reached the marketplace on schedule—multiphasic oral contraceptives, an injectable (Depo-Provera), and a subcutaneous progestin implant (Norplant). These had all been available for several years in many other countries. The four remaining methods mentioned in the report—improved ovulation-detection techniques, luteinizing hormone-releasing hormone (LHRH), prostaglandin analogues, and vaginal rings—are still being evaluated but are not yet available in the United States. The OTA report also listed eleven other methods as possible but doubtful. None of these is likely to become available in the foreseeable future, if ever.

Multiple products employing steroids are being studied for use by women. These include additional injectables and implants, estrogen gels, transdermal patches, vaginal suppositories, and sublingual tablets. In the area of barrier contraception, disposable diaphragms, previously approved but never marketed, are now again being researched. New spermicidal agents that may help to protect against the transmission of STDs are urgently being sought. Three vaccines are under investigation for immunization against STDs: human chorionic gonadotropin (hCG); a hormone from the zona pellucida (outer layer) of the ovum; and sperm. These are highly complex agents that require lengthy and expensive research, and they will probably be many years in development.

Meanwhile, the search continues for effective birth control methods for men, including substances such as male and female sex steroids, gossypol, and inhibin. These, too, are not expected to achieve widespread use for a number of years, if ever. In fact, the World Health Organization has recently estimated that it will be at least twenty years before a safe and reliable male contraceptive method becomes generally available. Two condoms, the minicondom (glans cap) and the bikini (panty) condom, were presented to the FDA's OB/GYN Device Panel in 1989; however, as there were no adequate data on safety and efficacy, neither of these was approved by the panel.

It is an unfortunate fact that individuals living outside the United States, including those in a number of developing countries, have access to a far wider array of contraceptives than do Americans. The current list includes a number of hormonal agents and several IUDs; also the Ovablock Plug is available in other countries for female sterilization. All of these methods are, in many ways, highly acceptable and potentially useful to either large numbers of people or to specific individuals because of their particular needs. However, it appears unlikely that most of these, or any other major changes in fertility-regulating technology, will soon become available to people living in the United States.

As in any field, there are certain prerequisites for major research and development activities. These necessarily include adequate funding and long-term commitment. Without both of these factors, it is impossible to recruit creative, innovative individuals to carry out the studies required to bring new technologies to the marketplace. The sad fact is that the amount of funding available for research in contraception has been progressively more limited in recent years. Any area that is perceived to be steadily less important and less academically and financially rewarding will clearly not attract the best and the brightest people. The general perception of the decreasing importance of contraceptive research and development has been reinforced by a steady decline in training grants, which further reduces the number of young researchers going into the field.

This decline began several years ago, probably for two key reasons. First, for a time, the pill and the IUD were considered to be close to ideal; therefore, the overall perception was that additional research was not really needed. At the same time, birth rates began to drop in many developed and some developing countries and the anxiety about a potential population explosion began to abate.

Unfortunately, neither of these perceptions has been proved correct, and there is no reason to feel at all sanguine about our current situation. Our contraceptive technology today, while infinitely superior to anything in the past, is still far from ideal. The population problem is getting steadily worse in many areas of the world, particularly in a number of developing countries. Although growth rates have slowed in a few countries, the ultimate solution to the population problem is many years down the road, and each year of delay in solving the problem will pose even greater difficulties with which future generations will have to contend.

In addition to training and sustained salary support, research efforts today demand increasing amounts of money. Progressively more expensive and more elaborate studies are needed for the development, FDA approval, and introduction of any new technology. Moreover, it is essential to continue to study the reproductive processes in both males and females to identify new ways in which to interfere, either temporarily or permanently, with some aspect of their function. Even having done so, the future development of any new fertility regulation methods resulting from these findings will be increasingly complex and expensive.

At the present time, the field is considerably underfunded and is totally unfunded by many groups previously engaged in contraceptive research. A number of past reviews of the subject have pointed out the importance of U.S. support. In 1969, 77 percent of all monies spent in this field came from the United States, up from 68 percent in 1964. Fifteen developed countries contributed 21 to 30 percent; approximately 2 percent came from developing countries. The same general pattern of funding has continued up to the present time. Thus, it is clear that the primary role in drug and device development still lies in those areas of the world that are more developed.

Funding Sources

Over the years, pharmaceutical companies, government agencies, universities, and nonprofit organizations have made major contributions to contraceptive research and development. Each of these groups has had its own specific and, in many cases, predictable mandates and agendas. Pharmaceutical companies have a major interest in the development of products that will be profitable for them and their shareholders. They are less inclined to support basic noncommercial-oriented research than are agencies in the public sector such as the National Institutes of Health, the U.S. Agency for International Development (AID), and universities.

Nonprofit groups, on the other hand, often have a stated commitment to research and training and thus are able to do basic work that would not be as appropriate for individuals working in the private sector. Organizations such as foundations are able to operate without the constraints that very often limit the focus of the activities of the other groups.

During the era of the development of oral contraceptives and IUDs, at least nine of the large U.S. pharmaceutical companies were carrying out research in the field of birth control. However, in the years since the end of that era, eight of these companies have stopped making major financial commitments to the field. There have been multiple reasons for this mass departure. They include the long time and high cost required for development and approval of new products, the limited time of exclusive marketing because of patent limitations, the escalating costs of product liability insurance, the increasing frequency of highly expensive litigation, and the pressures from anti–birth control groups in the United States.

Corporate decision making necessarily hinges on a satisfactory financial return on investments. Many companies, when trying to decide how best to use their available research-and-development funds, have recognized the relatively high cost and potentially low return of the study of new contraceptive agents. They have, therefore, increasingly put their monies into products that will cost less to develop and to obtain FDA approval, will produce less in the way of antagonism on the part of certain segments of society, and will be widely used. In this way, they guarantee a better return on their investments.

Many of the major pharmaceutical companies are based in developed countries that have aging and noncontracepting populations. Therefore, the current corporate goals often are to find products that will have long-term (and thus more profitable) use in the treatment of such things as cardiovascular disease and cancer. However, if certain of the constraints to contraceptive research and development were to be removed, some of the companies who have left the field might consider reentering, at least to some degree, the fertility-regulation arena.

Another outcome of these corporate decisions has been the establishment of at least a dozen smaller firms. The development and the promulgation of guidelines by the FDA for generic drugs have also expanded the number of those companies working in the field of contraception. These smaller companies' approaches are often quite different from those of the larger firms who used to do contraceptive research and development. In general, they have a single or only a few products into which they have put most of their available capital. Thus, it is critically important to them that they receive a profit from their investments in a reasonably short period of time. They are willing to assume a somewhat greater risk of liability to get quickly to the marketplace. They also have an additional special advantage; they are at far lower risk of boycott of their other products by groups opposed to contraception than are large companies that have developed products in many different therapeutic areas.

Multiple nonprofit organizations such as the Population Council, the Contraceptive Research and Development Program (CONRAD), Family Health International (FHI), the Program for Appropriate Technology in Health (PATH), and many universities have been involved in basic research and, in some instances, also the testing and marketing of new birth control techniques. In the past, organizations such as the Ford Foundation, the Rockefeller Foundation, and the Mellon Foundation have given considerable support to the field of contraception. International involvement continues, particularly through the World Health Organization. However, it has often been difficult to recruit and retain the highly qualified staff necessary for the development process, particularly for nonprofit and government groups where the salary expectations, both short- and long-term, are lower in general than they are in the private sector.

Fortunately, there has been gradually increasing recognition and acceptance of the fact that more effort and funding are urgently needed for the development and introduction of new contraceptive agents. One suggested approach is that additional government programs be established. For example, legislation has been introduced in Congress recommending the establishment of a number of new research centers. However, some people feel that the most effective use of funds might be to give additional support to organizations already working in the field.

Drug and Device Regulation

The organization responsible for making regulatory decisions in the United States is the U.S. Food and Drug Administration (FDA). Other countries, primarily those that are developed, also have regulatory bodies, varying in size and level of power. At the international level, the World Health Organization (WHO) has considerable input into drug development and evaluation.

The FDA has three major divisions with legislative jurisdiction over contraceptives. The first section deals with drugs, the second with medical devices, and the third with over-the-counter agents. In addition, it is responsible for the review of generic and "orphan" drugs (products used to treat specific uncommon diseases affecting only a small number of people and therefore never expected to be profitable).

In the past, new drugs were tested on human volunteers, often with insufficient regard for safety. There was not always proper communication by investigators about what the subjects might expect in terms of the possible benefits and adverse reactions from using a particular drug. For this reason, the FDA was established in this country in 1906 by the Pure Food and Drugs Act. As indicated by the name, it originally looked primarily at the misbranding of foods and drugs. Legislation passed in 1938 added a mandate to look at safety issues. Then, in 1962, an amendment was enacted in response to the thalidomide tragedy, giving the FDA much greater jurisdiction over efficacy issues.

Medical devices were added to the FDA purview in 1976 by the Medical Device Amendments, which required safety and efficacy data on each device prior to marketing. In 1984, the Drug Price Competition and Patent Restoration Act was passed by Congress. It was aimed at accelerating the approval of generic drugs and restored up to five years of patent time lost during the FDA approval process. Finally, in response to the need for products that protect against both pregnancy and STDs, new premarket guidelines for expedited approval were established in 1990.

While providing better protection to subjects, these laws also led to the development of extensive research protocols, some quite rational and others less so, that have added considerably to the time required for research and development and the expense involved. It was estimated in the mid-1990s that it cost approximately $150 million to bring a new contraceptive product to the marketplace, compared with the $50 to $55 million required in the mid-1970s. Current estimates have increased to $500 million and are projected to rise even more in the future. There are many steps involved in the development of a new drug or device, beginning with laboratory and animal studies. Only after the product has been found to be safe and effective in both these areas can human testing begin. Drug testing begins with a small number of volunteers and focuses primarily on safety, toxicity, and absorption (Phase one). The next round of studies is carried out using larger groups of individuals; these studies assess both safety and efficacy (Phase two). If these are successful, a third round of studies begins; these involve several hundred volunteers, carefully evaluating all aspects of their clinical course (Phase three).

The total time consumed in these trials varies from five to as many as fifteen or more years, depending on the particular product involved. The FDA review and approval process usually takes about two years but may be as long as seven or more years. If only conditional approval has been obtained, it is now more frequently required that further studies be carried out following marketing. These so-called postmarketing surveillance studies are important because it is often impossible to determine risks that have a very low incidence before there is widespread use of a product. Conversely, the same is also true of unanticipated and previously undocumented health benefits such as those seen with the use of the OCs.

To identify all significant new findings, the FDA has continued to require the reporting of adverse as well as beneficial experiences to the manufacturer and thus, in turn, to the FDA. In addition, the FDA has mandated the use of tracking registries for individual products when there are residual unresolved issues at the time of the conditional approval.

In recent years there have been concerns about the efficacy of the FDA in reviewing and approving new drugs and devices, as well as approving new indications for those already on the market. It has been well documented that new-product development is a very expensive and time-consuming endeavor; only one out of every ten thousand chemicals discovered in the laboratory ever makes it to the marketplace. Also, it is widely recognized that, although improved in recent years, there are still problems with regard to the FDA approval process. In some instances, FDA guidelines have been less than precise and consistent, and differences that arise between the FDA and the pharmaceutical industry are not always easily or quickly resolved. In addition, the FDA, in many cases, is constrained by legislative activity and impacted upon by congressional hearings and other forms of pressure often applied on the behalf of particular consumer groups. For example, congressional hearings have played a key role in family planning affairs—the oral contraceptives (the Nelson hearings) and the Contraceptive Vaginal Sponge (the Weiss hearings). In all probability, the Fountain hearings were a major factor in the FDA's continued refusal to approve Depo-Provera for so many years.

There are major variations in how individual countries regulate drugs and devices. The biggest problem for all regulatory agencies has always been determining the proper balance between the benefits and risks of any particular product. Work in the contraceptive field is particularly difficult and sensitive because it involves identifying agents that may be administered over considerable periods of time, and may, on occasion, also impact upon a developing fetus. Whereas a certain amount of risk can be tolerated when one is looking for drugs to be used in the treatment of a terminal malignancy, the amount of risk that is appropriate and acceptable for contraceptive agents is felt to be considerably less.

A natural consequence of the pressures applied to the FDA by certain consumer groups plus the constant awareness of the potential for congressional overview hearings is a tendency to be extremely cautious, to move very deliberately and to do nothing that could produce future problems. As a result the pace of formulating conclusions is frequently slow. Researchers must often deal with repeated alterations in preliminary protocols and multiple postponements of decisions regarding final study designs, all of which leads to delays in new drug and device approval.

The growing complexity of the FDA regulations has also created increasing difficulties in the development and approval process. Much of this has been necessary, but some observers do not believe that the FDA has always functioned as efficiently as it might. As already noted, a major reason for this is the fact that the agency is always in an extremely sensitive position. The media quickly pounces on any alleged adverse effects of drugs and devices, often without paying any attention to the fact that the findings are very preliminary in nature and are frequently based on statistically unproved data. Furthermore, due regard is not always given by the media to the relevance of animal data as it might possibly apply (or not apply) to humans. Finally, many people still fail to appreciate the fact that it is virtually impossible to create a product that is highly safe and effective and yet does not have at least a small potential for adverse effects in at least a small percentage of the population.

While the FDA has numerous consultant expert committees, these are almost all advisory in nature and may be (and on occasion have been) overruled at the discretion of the FDA. Moreover, although the FDA's legislative mandate is limited to the United States, its pronouncements have a very strong impact internationally: many developing countries do not have the funds or resources required to develop their own regulatory bodies and are almost totally dependent on agencies in the developed countries for evaluations of medical drugs and devices. This means that these agencies have an influence far beyond their own national borders and, in fact, are often both ethically and morally responsible for many of the medical development and approval processes throughout the whole world.

Stung by repeated attacks by the international medical community, the FDA has attempted to explain some of the differences in benefit/risk ratios between developed and developing countries. However, as in the case of DMPA, despite its recent belated approval, such explanations can never entirely dispel the perception on the part of some developing countries that they are receiving second-class medical care, good enough for their use but not good enough for people in the developed world.

Innovation Versus Liability

The legal climate in the United States continues to have a very direct and extremely negative impact on the development of new and innovative contraceptive drugs and devices in the United States—and also on the introduction of safe and effective products developed elsewhere in the world. Contraceptive research has been markedly hampered because of concerns about liability issues and the potential for future punitive damages against individuals and companies developing these newer technologies.

In recent years there has been a huge increase in the frequency and expense of litigation regarding contraceptive products. Liability costs for OCs are higher than for any other drug category. This situation has been spawned by the media's continued focus on adverse effects, by problems related to defective devices such as the Dalkon

Shield, and by the general perception that any contraceptive ought to have a very high level of effectiveness and virtually no risk. Another factor is that contraceptives are needed and used by a huge variety of individuals including those with serious health problems; however, these drugs are often erroneously perceived as being used almost entirely by healthy people. Therefore, the mandate has consistently been that they achieve a level of safety and efficacy rarely required of other products.

An additional complicating problem is the fact that these agents must be viewed from the perspective of at least three individuals—the person using the method, the sexual partner(s) and, coincidentally, a fetus that may result from failure or incorrect use of the method. This situation has led to an extremely conservative point of view on the part of the FDA, which places rigorous demands for documentation of both efficacy and safety on contraceptive products. Agents approved for marketing that have subsequently been found, upon wider use, to exhibit rare adverse side effects have put the FDA in a very defensive posture. Cynically put, it is easier not to approve a product than it is to face the potential for future conflict. Furthermore, once a contraceptive is on the market, almost any adverse effect, either related or even unrelated to the use of the product, can prove to be grounds for lucrative litigation.

Another major impact on fertility regulation comes from conservative groups—certain consumer and women's rights and self-help groups and extremists in the fundamentalist religious community. Often using litigation, these groups have been very influential in their demands on legislative bodies, regulatory agencies, and pharmaceutical companies. In fact, some of these groups have actually been quite successful in limiting the types of products that are selected for development and marketing in the United States. The ultimate impact of these outside forces is to restrict the available options to those they find acceptable. This necessarily excludes a considerable number of innovative drugs and devices already identified as useful or potentially useful.

A classic example of this situation has been the controversy surrounding antiprogesterones such as RU 486 (mifepristone). For many years, those interested in the study and use of these drugs as medical abortifacients have been unable to find a U.S. company willing to undertake the work necessary to move them toward FDA approval. Even more disturbing is the fact that the possibility was remote primarily because of the intense pressures, including threats of violence and plans to boycott all of the other products made by its developer, the French pharmaceutical company Roussel-Uclaf, and its German parent company Hoechst AG. These obstructive activities continued despite the fact that RU 486 had shown early promise as a contraceptive, a treatment for breast cancer, cervical softening before induction of labor, endometriosis, Cushing's syndrome, Addison's disease, glaucoma, premenstrual syndrome, and a number of cancers including unresectable meningiomas of the brain. The greatest hope for the antiprogesterones and similar products has been that they may start to have an impact on the two hundred thousand deaths from unsafe abortions that occur each year; in some countries, these deaths account for almost half of the total maternal mortality.

Despite the approval of RU 486 by France and Great Britain (and its probable approval by China, Holland, and some of the Scandinavian countries), pressure in the United States effectively blocked the study and use of RU 486. In fact, the U.S. State Department implied in 1981 that it might reconsider its support of World Bank activities if any funds were being used by WHO for its international clinical trials of RU 486. Also, WHO expressed concerns that the United States would stop funding all of its programs if it continued its studies of RU 486. As a result of all of these obstructions, this agent did not receive final FDA approval until September 2000. It is currently marketed as Mifeprex™. A further complication has been the vigorous attempt on the part of the company making Cytotec™ (misoprostol), a drug used for many years in the treatment of ulcers, to distance itself from the RU 486 debate, since it is used, with FDA approval, as the second part of the two-day regimen to induce early medical abortions.

In many instances, the decision making as to whether or not to pursue a particular line of research or product development has shifted from the medical to the marketing and legal divisions of pharmaceutical companies. This is not unexpected, given the number of adverse legal decisions in recent years made without the benefit of any scientific evidence such as the cases leading to the demise of most of the IUDs, the near-demise of Norplant, and the bankrupting of Dow Corning over the issue of silicone gel-filled breast implants.

One of the most flagrant abuses of legal power was a $5,151,030 award made in a case alleging fetal damage from the use of the spermicide Ortho-Gynol, based on a single badly flawed article in the medical literature. This decision was handed down by a judge in Georgia in 1985 despite overwhelming medical evidence to the contrary, and for a time the repercussions threatened the very existence of spermicidal agents. Multiple studies before and after the trial pointed out that no such association existed. In fact, two of the coauthors of the cited paper have since publicly retracted their original conclusions and have questioned the wisdom of their publication of the article.

Even those cases that are successfully defended may have a major negative impact on public opinion, often leading to a decrease in a company's sales or, as in the case of the IUD, actual removal of FDA-approved products from the marketplace. All of these factors taken together have tended to limit the commitment of time, money, and effort to a field that is generally perceived to be at high risk for litigation and therefore potentially offers a relatively poor return on corporate investment.

Political Considerations

Politics and political interventions have also played key roles in the contraceptive research and development process. Congressional committee hearings have been increasingly important in determining patterns of drug and device approval. As a result, high-level officials at the FDA have had to spend considerable time testifying before these committees. Often these officials do not consider this to be time well spent, and some even feel that it has been counterproductive.

In the field of contraception, virtually no major technique has escaped the public onus of a congressional hearing. These hearings have increased public concern about the safety and effectiveness of the contraceptive in question and the requirements for its approval. In addition, "drug lag" has caused confrontations between the FDA and many individuals (including congressmen) who were worried about the slowness of the research-and-development and approval processes. Finally, extensive documentation now exists regarding the adverse interaction between monumental damage awards and cost-prohibitive product liability policies and procedures. Congress, a high percentage of whose members are attorneys with close political fiscal ties, has continued to be reluctant to enact any legislation directly addressing this major problem, including such possible solutions as tort reform and limitations on pain and suffering awards.

It has been noted by several observers that the congressional overview of FDA activities has, on occasion, actually slowed the progress of drug development. Over the years, there has been an increased watch-dog attitude often stimulated by groups with their own particular agendas in mind. Also, in recent years, there has been a notable lack of congressional support for the FDA; in fact, there has been a curtailment of some of the organization's resources.

In some instances, political pressures rather than scientific data appear to have mandated the outcome of FDA decisions. The classic example, as already noted, has been the fact that for more than twenty years the FDA refused to approve DPMA as a contraceptive agent, despite the unanimous recommendations of its own advisory committees to do so, and the fact that it was being used safely and effectively by millions of women in more than ninety other countries. There is no doubt that, to some degree, this decision was strongly influenced by the congressional hearings on this subject, resulting from major efforts spent to block its approval by certain feminist and consumer groups.

The Doctor-Patient Relationship

It is impossible to look at the overall contraceptive scene without recognizing that a major part of this scenario lies in the changing relationship between physicians and their patients, particularly women. There is a growing feeling among consumers that medical care should provide immediate and complete solutions to their problems. When this does not occur (which is obviously inevitable in many situations), there is an increasing tendency to turn to the courts for a resolution. This has resulted in a progressive erosion of the doctor-patient relationship, escalating costs of medical malpractice insurance, and rapidly expanding health-care expenses as more and more physicians have felt compelled to practice defensive medicine. Thus, in an effort to protect themselves, doctors often order unindicated and unnecessary x-rays and laboratory tests. Increasingly they are trying to avoid offering health care to women perceived to be at high risk for medical complications and/or for instituting lawsuits.

This has led, for example, to a dramatic and steady decline in the availability of obstetrical care, particularly for women in rural areas and those in lower socio-economic groups. Unfortunately, surveys have shown that 60 percent of doctors who used to practice obstetrics will no longer accept pregnant women as patients. This situation is now also being seen among nurse practitioners, as their insurance costs go up and their liability increases. Concerns about possible litigation have also led to poor utilization of existing methods of contraception in the United States as compared to other countries. Regarding the IUD, for example, physicians continue to fear complications and lawsuits, despite good medical and legal evidence to the contrary.

Once a particular attitude has been progressively embedded over a period of time, it then moves into a position of cultural acceptability. In previous times, the instituting of lawsuits against physicians and/or pharmaceutical companies was rare. However, as this practice became more and more common, it became culturally acceptable. Now it is an accepted norm for behavior in this particular area.

Finally, very often the initial discussion between a physician and a patient about contraception fails to deal with some of the underlying psychological considerations that should be explored. This is increasingly true now that the time allowed for patient care is being progressively limited. Unless the conversation goes beyond the superficialities of the available contraceptive techniques, certain patient attitudes may escape notice and the result may well be poor adherence to the chosen method. Failure and discontinuation rates are often unnecessarily high because of misunderstandings on the part of women, particularly teenagers, stemming from the lack of appropriate dialogues between them and their health-care providers.

The Loss of the U.S. Leadership Role

Between 1965 and 1974, a period that has often been called the decade of contraceptive growth, there was an ever-increasing amount of money going into reproductive research. This resulted in great improvements in our contraceptive technology. Although contributions to this effort came from many countries, by and large the United States was the leader in both basic science research and contraceptive development. The United States also provided much of the training of both scientists and health-care providers from developing countries and was a major source of support to many international family planning programs.

Unfortunately, in recent years, the United States has lost its leadership role in this field. Increasingly, contraceptive development is being carried out in other countries—although, ironically, often with U.S. dollars. This is particularly true in the case of new and innovative agents where the potential for risk in the United States is now perceived to far exceed the potential for profit. As a result, American-based companies are now spending an increasingly higher percentage of their research and development dollars overseas. Even more distressing is the fact that fewer and fewer of those products that are found to have real potential are being returned to the United States for further study and eventual application for FDA approval. Thus, many of the products resulting from this research are not—and may never be—available to U.S. women.

The overall result has been the U.S. failure to develop and/or introduce any new and innovative methods of contraception for more than twenty years, with the exception of the subdermal implants and possibly the vaginal pouch. Unless this situation changes, Americans in the twenty-first century are going to have no methods of family planning that are significantly better than the ones that were available during the twentieth century.

12

The Future of Contraception

THERE IS A clear need for new and improved contraceptive methods. Many people do not fully grasp the importance of fertility regulation, and the resources being put into this field continue to decline. The regulatory process is slow and expensive, and product liability and medical malpractice insurance, as well as lawsuits, have proved to be major stumbling blocks to the development of new and better contraceptive agents. Finally, public and private agencies, corporations, and institutional review boards (IRBs) of major universities are more and more reluctant to approve studies because of their concerns about possible liability.

The problem in the United States today is multifaceted. Resolution of only one aspect such as low funding would provide a much improved climate for a renewed interest in contraceptive research and development. However, maximum impact will only come when there has been considerable improvement in most or all of the areas this book has identified as impediments to the development, approval, and marketing of new products that are safer, more effective, and more acceptable than those currently available.

A number of interesting research projects are currently underway that could have salutary effects in the future, given sufficient funding. Oral contraceptives might be improved in a number of ways while still maintaining their high levels of efficacy, safety, and health benefits. The hormonal agents now used in the OCs and new ones currently in development could be employed in a variety of different formulations and methods of administration, improving the ease of use, effectiveness, safety, acceptability, and duration of action. Such techniques include gels, injectables, implants, sublingual and vaginal tablets, biodegradable microcapsules, contraceptive bracelets, and nasal sprays. Interesting preliminary evidence shows that OCs using melatonin in place of estrogen might actually decrease the risk of breast cancer.

Ovulation predication and confirmation might be made much more practical and useful. IUDs might be made even safer and more effective by the addition of metals, hormones, or other chemical agents to new or existing devices. Studies on a number of new means of not only suppressing ovulation but also blocking the development of sperm are underway. Finally, menses inducers—agents to be given once a month at the time of expected menses—are another area of ongoing research.

Newer and more acceptable forms of barrier contraception are also under study, including improved spermicidal and anti-STD agents. Research is being conducted in an attempt to find male contraceptive techniques that can be administered orally, by injection, or by implantation. Improvements in both male and female sterilization techniques are possible. It has been shown that if these procedures were to be made predictably and reliably reversible, this approach would be more popular. Moreover, with better patient selection and improved procedural methods, there would likely be fewer requests for reversal. Considerably further down the road is the use of vaccines that could block one part of a woman's reproductive process or, alternatively, some portion of the male's contribution to the establishment of a pregnancy.

Just as important, if not more so, is the need to find ways to encourage better use of our current birth control methods. There are many myths about the existing safe and effective methods. The result is that American contraceptive utilization is well below that of other countries. For example, the risks of OCs have been exaggerated; newer data on low-dose pills should be widely distributed to put them into better perspective as a very safe option for most women. The current poorly documented fear of breast cancer should be countered by the very well-documented reduction in the risks of endometrial and ovarian cancers as well as the reduction in the total lifetime probability of developing any malignancy with OC use.

IUDs have suffered an even more disastrous fate of underutilization. Acceptance and use rates are low, due primarily to exaggerated fears about infection. This issue should be put to rest; and the long-term benefits of IUD use should be promoted. In addition, it is important that IUDs be recognized as contraceptives, not abortifacients.

Better utilization will also depend on improving consumer communication and understanding, starting with sex education in our nation's schools. Media of all types—newspaper, magazines, television, and radio—could be of great assistance and should be encouraged to join in the fight against unplanned pregnancy and STDs. Unfortunately, all forms of media, particularly television, have been counterproductive, using sex not only in entertainment programming but also in the promotion of all sorts of products. Only rarely are contraception, STD transmission, and unwanted pregnancies mentioned.

One stunning example of media irresponsibility concerns the American College of Obstetricians and Gynecologists (ACOG). The organization tried several years ago to place a public service message on TV aimed at encouraging the use of contraceptives by sexually active teenagers. All the major networks refused ACOG, claiming that the spots were too suggestive and provocative—too controversial to run. Finally, under pressure they reversed their decisions—provided that the word *contraception* was not mentioned!

Hopefully the current moves toward improved health care, particularly for women, and concerns about population and the environment will be of help in these matters. Given the present disheartening disenchantment with today's contraceptive technology and the decrease in funding for the development of new and improved drugs and devices, it is imperative that agencies of all types begin to apply part of their resources to this essential field of scientific endeavor. There is still an urgent need for individuals to be able to control their fertility safely, effectively, and acceptably. In view of the enormity of our current medical and socioeconomic problems, and the tremendous potential of current and projected research, it would indeed be foolhardy and shortsighted to deny a portion of the world's resources to contraceptive research and development and to the improved utilization of current methods.

Epilogue

WOMEN TODAY HAVE a greater risk of dying with a full-term pregnancy than they have with the use of any of the currently available contraceptive methods. It is extremely unfortunate that there are so many misunderstandings about the various birth control techniques and their risk/benefit ratios. It is very important that women and their health-care providers stay up-to-date on all the forms of contraception—their advantages and disadvantages—and to have a clear understanding of the options. For many years, American women have been found to be poor users of the available birth control methods; the result has been an alarming number of unplanned and often unwanted pregnancies as well as millions of induced abortions.

Because of the growing recognition of our deteriorating contraceptive research and development situation, a number of critical reviews have served to pinpoint some of the most important contributory factors. Key among these is the steady decline in the amount of funding available from both the public and private sectors. There has been a marked decrease in the amount of pharmaceutical company activity. Only one or two major U.S. firms are currently engaged in active contraceptive research and development, whereas there used to be at least nine such companies. In addition, there has been a loss of interest in working in this field. It is no longer perceived to be a viable career opportunity.

An additional important factor has been the increasingly litigious climate in the United States; it has had a direct and very negative impact on all aspects of contraceptive development and usage. Still another major facet of the problem is the long and expensive regulatory process the FDA requires for new drugs and devices to reach the marketplace. Finally, as fertility regulation is involved with two highly sensitive areas—that of human sexuality and reproduction—it was almost inevitable that certain segments of our society would begin to focus on this field to both its short- and long-term detriment.

There are several major reasons for improving contraception utilization. First, to reach her maximum potential, a woman must be able to plan her pregnancies. This is particularly important for American teenagers who now have the dubious distinction of having the highest pregnancy and abortion rates in the developed world. On a much broader scale, it is essential that people be able to curtail their unwanted fertility, as we are fast using up our nonrenewable resources and producing gross contamination of our environment. Finally, rampant population growth is now recognized to be the major source of many of our most severe and unresolved problems.

While there are some residual difficulties with all of our currently available contraceptive methods, particularly in the area of adverse side effects, some of the newer techniques now under investigation may help to rectify this situation. In the meantime, it is essential that all women recognize that very safe and effective methods of birth control already exist. It is vital for a woman who does not wish to become pregnant to learn about these methods, to select the best one for her, and to use it consistently until such time as she decides to have a baby.

Suggested Reading

Chapter 2

Carpenter, S., L. S. Neinstein. 1986. Weight gain in adolescent and young adult oral contraceptive users. *J. Adol. Health Care* 7:342–344.

Clarkson, T. B., M. R. Adams, J. R. Kaplan, et al. 1989. From menarche to menopause: coronary artery atherosclerosis and protection in cynomolgus monkeys. *Am. J. Obstet. Gynecol.* 160:1280–1285.

Colditz, G. A., and The Nurses' Health Study Research Group. 1994. Oral contraceptive use and mortality during 12 years of follow-up: The Nurses' Health Study. *Ann. Intern. Med.* 120:821–826.

DeCherney, A. 1996. Bone-sparing properties of oral contraceptives. *Am. J. Obstet. Gynecol.* 174:15–20.

Delbanco, S. F., J. Mauldon, M. D. Smith. 1997. Little knowledge and limited practice: emergency contraceptive pills, the public, and the obstetrician-gynecologist. *Obstet. Gynecol.* 89: 1006–1011.

Fotherby, K., A. D. S. Caldwell. 1994. New progestogens in oral contraception. *Contraception* 49:1–32.

Grimes, D. A., E. G. Raymond, B. S. Jones. 2001. Emergency contraception over the counter: the medical and legal imperatives. *JAMA* 98:151–155.

Peterson, H. B., N. C. Lee. 1989. The health effects of oral contraceptives: misperceptions, controversies, and continuing good news. *Clin. Obstet. Gynecol.* 32:339–355.

Petitti, D. B., S. Sidney, C. P. Quesenberry. 1998. Oral contraceptive use and myocardial infarction. *Contraception* 57:143–155.

Stewart, F. H., C. C. Harper, C. E. Ellertson, et al. 2001. Clinical breast and pelvic examination requirements for hormonal contraception: current practice vs. evidence. *JAMA* 285:2232–2239.

Thomas, D. B. 1991. Oral contraceptives and breast cancer: review of the epidemiological literature. In *Oral Contraceptives and Breast Cancer*. Committee on the Relationship Between Oral Contraceptives and Breast Cancer. Institute of Medicine, Division of Health Promotion and Disease Prevention. Washington, D.C.: National Academy Press.

Chapter 3

Frank, M. L., A. N. Poindexter, L. M. Cornin, et al. 1993. One-year experience with subdermal contraceptive implants in the United States. *Contraception* 48:229–243.

Shoupe, D., D. R. Mishell. 1989. NORPLANT®: subdermal implant system for long-term contraception. *Am. J. Obstet. Gynecol.* 160:1286–1292.

Wehrle, K. E. 1994. The NORPLANT® System: easy to insert, easy to remove. *Nurse Practitioner* 19(4):47–54.

Chapter 4

Lande, R. E. 1995. New era for injectables. *Population Reports* 23 (August): 2.

Mainwaring R., H. A. Hales, K. Stevenson, et al. 1995. Metabolic parameter, bleeding and weight changes in U.S. women using progestin only contraceptives. *Contraception* 51:149–153.

Skegg, D. C. G., E. A. Noonan, C. Paul, et al. 1995. Depot medroxyprogesterone acetate and breast cancer. A pooled analysis of the World Health Organization and New Zealand studies. *JAMA* 273:799–804.

Chapter 5

Farley, T. M. M., M. J. Rosenberg, P. Rowe, et al. 1992. Intrauterine devices and pelvic inflammatory disease: an international perspective. *Lancet* 339:785–788.

Forrest, J. D. 1994. Acceptability of IUDs in the United States. In Bardin, C. W., D. R. Mishell Jr., eds. Proceedings from the Fourth International Conference on IUDs. Butterworth-Heinemann, 90–99.

Grimes, D. A. 1992. The intrauterine device, pelvic inflammatory disease, and infertility: the confusion between hypothesis and knowledge. *Fertil. Steril.* 58:670–673.

Mastroianni, L., Jr. 1997. No evidence to support intrauterine contraceptive device and embryo destruction. *Am. J. Obstet. Gynecol.* 172:981. Letter.

Piccinino, L. J., W. D. Mosher. 1998. Trends in contraceptive use in the United States: 1982–1995. *Fam. Plann. Perspect.* 30:4–10, 46.

Sivin, I. 1989. IUDs are contraceptives, not abortifacients: a comment on research and belief. *Stud. Fam. Plann.* 20:355–359.

Trieman, K., L. Liskin, A. Kols, et al. IUDs—an update. Population Reports Series B, no. 5, Baltimore, Johns Hopkins School of Public Health Population Information Program, December 1995.

Chapter 6

Cates, W., K. M. Stone. 1992. Family planning, sexually transmitted disease, and contraceptive choice: a literature update. *Fam. Plann. Perspect.* 24:75–84.

Centers for Disease Control and Prevention. 1993. Update: barrier protection against HIV infection and other sexually transmitted diseases. *MMWR* 42:589–591, 597.

Trussell, J., K. Sturgen, J. Strickler, et al. 1994. Comparative contraceptive efficacy of the female condom and other barrier methods. *Fam. Plann. Perspect.* 26:66–72.

Chapter 7

Ryder, B., H. Campbell. 1995. Natural family planning in the 1990s. *Lancet* 346:233.

Wilcox, A. J., C. R. Weionberg, D. D. Baird. 1995. Timing of sexual intercourse in relation to ovulation. Effects on the probability of contraception, survival of the pregnancy, and sex of the baby, *New Engl. J. Med.* 333:1517.

Chapter 8

Kolata, G. 1974. !Kung hunter-gathers: feminism, diet and birth control, *Science* 185:932.

Thapa, S., R. V. Short, M. Potts. 1988. Breastfeeding, birthspacing and their effects on child survival. *Nature* 335:679.

Chapter 9

Mishell, D. R., Jr. 1993. Vaginal contraceptive rings. *Ann. Med.* 25:191–197.

Peterson, H. B., Z. Xia, J. M. Hughes, et al. 1996. The risk of pregnancy after tubal sterilization: findings from the U.S. Collaborative Review of Sterilization. *Am. J. Obstet. Gynecol.* 174: 1161–1170.

Wilcox, L. S., B. Martinez-Schnell, H. B. Peterson, et al. 1992. Menstrual function after tubal sterilization. *Am. J. Epidemiol.* 135:1368–1381.

Chapter 10

Frezieres, R. G., T. L. Walsh, A. L. Nelson, et al. 1999. Evaluation of the efficacy of a polyurethane condom: results from a randomized, controlled clinical trial. *Fam. Plann. Perspect.* 31:81–87.
Manson, J. E., P. M. Ridker, A. Spelsberg, et al. 1999. Vasectomy and subsequent cardiovascular disease in U.S. physicians. *Contraception* 59:181–186.

Chapter 11

American College of Obstetricians and Gynecologists. "Poll shows women still skeptical of contraceptive safety" (press release). Washington, DC: ACOG, January 20, 1994.
Peipert, J. F., J. Gutmann. 1993. Oral contraceptive risk assessment: a survey of 247 educated women. *Obstet. Gynecol.* 82:112–117.

Chapter 12

Centers for Disease Control and Prevention. 1999. Achievements in public health, 1900–1999: family planning. *MMWR* 48: 1073–1080.
Institute of Medicine. Contraceptive Research and Development: Looking to the Future. Washington, D.C.: National Academy Press, 1996.

General

Brown, Sarah S., and Leon Eisenberg. *The Best Intentions: Unintended Pregnancy and the Well-Being of Children and Families.* Washington D.C.: National Academy Press, 1995.
Djerassi, Carl. *The Politics of Contraception.* New York: W.W. Norton & Company, 1979.

Finch, B. E., and Hugh Green. *Contraception Through the Ages.* Springfield, Ill.: Charles C. Thomas, 1963.

Haseltine, Florence P., and Beverly G. Jacobson. *Women's Health Research: A Medical and Policy Primer.* Washington, D.C.: Health Press International, 1997.

Mastroianni, Luigi, Jr., Peter J. Donaldson, and Thomas T. Kane. *Developing New Contraceptives: Obstacles and Opportunities.* Washington, D.C.: National Academy Press, 1990.

Potts, Malcolm, and Roger Short. *Ever Since Adam and Eve: The Evolution of Human Sexuality.* Cambridge: Cambridge University Press, 1999.

Skuy, Percy. *Tales of Contraception.* Ontario: Janssen-Ortho Inc., 1995.

Index

Abortion, 75
  ancient methods of, 8
  in Sweden, 18
Abstinence. *See* Periodic abstinence
Acne, oral contraceptives and,
  43–45, 75
Adrenal glands, oral contraceptives
  and, 41
Age, oral contraceptives and, 75
AIDS. *See* HIV/AIDS
Albert the Great, 1
Aldridge method of sterilization,
  200
Alzheimer's disease, oral
  contraceptives and, 35
Amenorrhea
  clinical management of, 69–70
  oral contraceptives and, 75
American College of Obstetricians
  and Gynecologists (ACOG),
  240
Anemia, oral contraceptives and,
  75–76
Antibiotics, oral contraceptives and,
  75
Antimicrobials, oral contraceptives
  and, 76

Anxiety states, oral contraceptives
  and, 76
Atherosclerosis, oral contraceptives
  and, 76–77
Avicenna, 4–5, 6, 136

Barrier contraceptives, 166–67
  cervical caps, 175–78
  diaphragms, 171–75
  female condoms, 182–84
  resuming use of, 194
  spermicides, 168–71
  vaginal contraceptive sponges,
  178–82
Biliary tract, oral contraceptives
  and, 40
Billings method, for periodic
  abstinence, 187–88
Bird folklore, about fertility, 2
Bleeding
  clinical management of, 68–69
  intrauterine devices and, 148–49
  new injectables for controlling,
  133
  women's attitudes toward, 126–27
Bleeding disorders, oral
  contraceptives and, 77

Blood coagulation, oral
    contraceptives and, 47
Breast cancer
    injectable contraceptives and,
        128–29
    oral contraceptives and, 32,
        65–68, 77
Breast-feeding. *See also* Lactational
    amenorrhea
    fertility rates and, 192
    HIV/AIDs transmission and, 196
Breasts
    clinical management of changes
        in, 70–71
    oral contraceptives and, 39

Calendar method, for periodic
    abstinence, 186
Cancer, injectable contraceptives
    and, 128–29
Candidiasis (moniliasis), oral
    contraceptives and, 50
Carbohydrates, oral contraceptives
    and, 54–55
Cardiovascular disease, 80–81
    oral contraceptives and, 52–54
Casanova, Giovanni Giacomo, 5
Case control studies, 59
Castor oil plant, 7
Category I conditions (WHO rating
    scale), 74
Category II conditions (WHO
    rating scale), 74
Category III conditions (WHO
    rating scale), 74
Category IV conditions (WHO
    rating scale), 74
Central nervous system, oral
    contraceptives' effect on, 41–43
Cervical cancer, barrier
    contraceptives and, 167
Cervical caps, 175–76
    advantages of, 177–78
    disadvantages of, 178
    effectiveness of, 176
    safety of, 177
    types of, 175–76
    using, 176–77

Cervical mucus method, for
    periodic abstinence, 187–88
Cervix, oral contraceptives and,
    36–37
Chang, Min-Chueh, 11
Chastity belts, 7
Chlamydia trachomatis, oral
    contraceptives and, 50
Chloasma, oral contraceptives and,
    45–46, 78
Cholesterol, 52–54
Christian, Donald, 141
Cleopatra, queen of Egypt, 3
Coagulation, oral contraceptives
    and, 47
Cohort studies, 59
Coitus, contraceptive techniques at
    time of, 6
Coitus interruptus, 6, 206–9. *See
    also* Male contraception
Coitus reservatus, 6
Coitus saxonicus, 6
Collaborative Review of
    Sterilization (CREST), 201–3
Colorectal cancer, 35
Colton, Frank, 11
Combined pills, 16
Condoms, 5, 25–26
    female, 182–84
    male. *See* Condoms, male
Condoms, male, 5, 194, 209–10
    advantages of, 212
    disadvantages, 212
    effectiveness of, 212–13
    types of, 210–11
    using, 211–12
Contraception. *See also*
    Contraception, male;
    Pregnancies
    folklore about, 1–2
    future of, 238–40
    improving utilization of, 242
    need for better, 220–22
    pessaries for preventing, 4
Contraception, male, 223. *See also*
    Contraception
    immunological methods for, 218
    medical approaches to, 215–18

Contraceptive gels, 199
Contraceptive patches, 198–99
Contraceptive research and
    development, 222–25
    funding for, 225–27
    litigation and, 231–34
    loss of U.S. leadership role in,
        237
    political considerations and,
        234–35
Contraceptive sponges, 178–82
Contraceptive vaccines, 204
Contraceptives
    barrier. *See* Barrier contraceptives
    emergency. *See* Emergency
        contraceptives
    implant. *See* Implants,
        contraceptive
    injectable. *See* Injectable
        contraceptives
    oral. *See* Oral contraceptives
    at time of coitus, 6
Counseling, for oral contraceptive
    users, 93–94
Cramping, intrauterine devices and,
    148
CREST (Collaborative Review of
    Sterilization), 201–3
Cu-7 intrauterine devices, 139–40,
    161
Cyclo-Provera. *See* Lunelle
Cyclofem. *See* Lunelle

Dalkon Shield, 141–42, 161
Depo-Provera (DMPA), 118–22
    administrating, 122–23
    advantages of, 123–25, 132–33
    bleeding patterns and, 125–26
    cancer and, 128–29
    contraindications for, 131
    disadvantages of, 127–28
    discontinuation rates of, 132
    effectiveness of, 123
    fetal effects of, 131
    future fertility and, 130–31
    for lactating women, 195
Depression, 78
    oral contraceptives and, 41–42

DES (diethylstilbestrol), 79, 100
Diabetes, 78–79
Diaphragms, 171–72
    advantages of, 174
    disadvantages of, 174–75
    effectiveness of, 172–73
    safety of, 174
    types of, 172
    using, 173–74
Diethylstilbestrol (DES), 79, 100
Diosgenin, 10
Djerassi, Carl, 11
DMPA. *See* Depo-Provera (DMPA)
Doctor-patient relationships, 235–37
Douching, 203–4
Drospirenon, 105
Dumas cap, 175
Dysmenorrhea, 79

Ears, effects of oral contraceptives
    on, 48
Ectopic pregnancy, 79
Eggs, 186–87
Emergency Contraceptive
    Connection, 104–5
Emergency contraceptives, 99–105
Emotional approaches, for
    unwanted pregnancies, 6–7
Endocrine glands, oral
    contraceptives and, 41
Endometrial cancer, 31–32
Endometriosis, 33, 79
Estradiol, 10
Estrogen, in oral contraceptives, 13
Estrogen-dependent tumors, 80
Estrogens, 10
Eurilthas, 8
Expulsion problems, intrauterine
    devices and, 149–50
Eyes, effects of oral contraceptives
    on, 47–48

Fallopian tubes, effects of oral
    contraceptives on, 38
Family history, 80
FDA (Food and Drug
    Administration), 227–31
Fellner, Otfried Otto, 10

Female barrier contraceptives. *See*
    Barrier contraceptives
Female condoms, 182–84. *See also*
    Condoms; Condoms, male
Female sterilization, 199–203
FemCap, 176
Fertility
    folklore about, 1–2
    return of, 91–92
Fertility rates, breast-feeding and,
    192
Fetus, oral contraceptives on, 92–93
Folklore, about fertility, 1–2
Food and Drug Administration
    (FDA), 227–31

G. D. Searle & Company, 13
Gallbladder, effects of oral
    contraceptives on, 40
Gallbladder disease, 80
Garcia, Celso-Ramon, 13
Gastrointestinal tract, oral
    contraceptives and, 39–40
Gels, contraceptive, 199
Goldzieher, Joseph W., 13
Gossypol, 217
Gräfenberg, Ernest, 137
Gyne T intrauterine devices, 140

Haberlandt, Ludwig, 10
Hair loss, oral contraceptives and,
    46
HDL (high-density lipoprotein), 52
Headaches
    clinical management of, 71–73
    oral contraceptives and, 80
Heart disease. *See* Cardiovascular
    disease
High-density lipoprotein (HDL), 52
Hippocrates, 3, 7, 136
Hirsutism, 81
HIV/AIDS transmission, 81
    barrier contraceptives and, 167
    breast-feeding and, 196
    contraceptive implants and,
        113–14
    oral contraceptive use and, 49

Hoagland, Hudson, 11
Human papillomavirus (HPV), 36
Hypertension, 81–82
    oral contraceptives and, 62–64

Ibis, fertility and, 2
Immune systems, oral
    contraceptives on, 48
Immunologic methods, for
    contraception, 204
Implanon, 116
Implants, contraceptive, 107–8
    advantages of, 111–12
    candidates for, 112–13
    continuation rates of, 112
    counseling for, 113–14
    disadvantages of, 112
    future of, 116–17
    inserting, 109–10
    for lactating women, 195
    litigation over, 114–16
    removing, 110
    side effects of, 111
Infectious mononucleosis, 82
Infertility, 2
Infibulation, 7–8
Injectable contraceptives, 118–22.
    See also Depo-Provera (DMPA)
    administrating, 122–23
    advantages of, 123–25
    bleeding patterns and, 125–26
    cancer and, 128–29
    disadvantages of, 127–28
    effectiveness of, 123
    future fertility and, 130–31
    monthly, 133–34
    new regimens of, 133–35
Intrauterine devices (IUDs), 26, 240
    advantages of, 155–56
    cramping and bleeding symptoms
        for, 148–49
    Cu-7, 139–40, 161
    current, 138–41
    current types of, 138–41
    Dalkon Shield episode and,
        141–42
    development of, 136–38

disadvantages of, 156
effectiveness of, 144
expulsion problems with, 149–50
fetal damage and, 153
future, 164–65
good candidates for using,
    156–57
history of, 136
insertion procedures for, 146–47
insertion techniques for, 144–45
insertion time for, 145–46
instructions for using, 158–59
lost tails and, 151–52
malignancy and, 155
mechanisms of action of, 142–44
multiload, 140
myths and misperceptions about,
    160
pelvic inflammatory disease and,
    153–55
perforation problems with,
    150–51
poor candidates for using, 157–58
pregnancy diagnosis and, 152–53
removal of, 147–48
resuming use of, 194–95
usage, 161–64
Irving method of sterilization, 200
Ismail the Bloodthirsty, 205
IUDs. *See* Intrauterine devices
    (IUDs)

Kabuta-Gata, 5
Karezza, 6
Kong Fou, 6
Koolpi, 8
Kroener method of sterilization,
    200

Lactation, 82
    using oral contraceptives during,
    195
Lactational amenorrhea, 192–93
    effectiveness of, 193–94
LDL (low-density lipoprotein), 52
Lea Shield diaphragms, 172

Leeuwenhoek, Antonie van, 8, 185
Levonorgestrel, 101–2
Levonorgestrel butanoate, 133
Levonorgestrel
    cyclobutylcarboxylate, 133
Libido, oral contraceptives and, 42
Lipids, 52–54, 83
Lippes, Jack, 138
Lippes Loops intrauterine device,
    159
Liver, oral contraceptives and, 40
Liver disease, 83
Low-density lipoprotein (LDL), 52
Lunelle, 134
Lung disease, 83

"M" intrauterine devices, 139
McCormick, Kathryn Dexter, 12
Madlener method of sterilization,
    200
Majzlin Spring, 139
Male condoms. *See* Condoms, male
Male continence, 6
Male contraception, 206–9
Male sterilization, 199, 213–15
Malignancies, intrauterine devices
    and, 155
Malignant melanoma, oral
    contraceptives and, 45
Marguilies Coil, 138, 139
Marker, Russell E., 10–11
Mastroianni, Luigi, 12
Meclizine, 101
Medical devices, 228
Menses, perceptions of role of, 2–3
Menstrual problems, 32–33
    oral contraceptives and, 51
Mesigyna, 134
Migraine headaches, clinical
    management of, 72
Minerals, oral contraceptives and,
    47
Minipills, 16, 97–99
    for lactating women, 195
Mittelschmerz, 33, 84
Moniliasis (candidiasis), oral
    contraceptive and, 50

Monophasic oral contraceptives, 105
Monthly injectable contraceptives, 133–34
Morning-after pill. *See* Emergency contraceptives
Moroccan revenge, 7
Multiload intrauterine devices, 140
Multiphasic oral contraceptives, 105
Musculoskeletal system, oral contraceptives and, 46
Myocardial infarction, risk of, 62
Myths, about oral contraceptives, 93–94

Natural family planning. *See* Periodic abstinence
Nausea, clinical management of, 70
Norethindrone, 11
Noristerat, 133
Norplant II, 116
Norplant System, 107–8
    advantages of, 111–12
    candidates for, 112–13
    continuation rates of, 112
    counseling for, 113–14
    disadvantages of, 112
    litigation over, 114–16
    side effects of, 111
Nose, oral contraceptives and, 48
Nova T intrauterine devices, 140
NuvaRing, 198

Obesity, oral contraceptives and, 84
Oneida Community, 6
Oral contraceptives, 4. *See also* Progestin-only pills (POPs); specific medical condition
    adverse effects of, 60–68
    age issues and, 20–22
    ancient methods of, 6–7
    assessing side effects of, 57–60
    biliary tract and, 40
    blood coagulation and, 47
    breast cancers and, 32, 65–68, 77
    breasts and, 39
    carbohydrates and, 54–55

choosing particular, 23–24
clinical management of side effects of, 68–73
compliance and continuation of use, 95–97
counseling and, 93–94
ears and, 48
effectiveness of, 19–20
endocrine glands and, 41
evaluating studies of side effects of, 55–57
eyes and, 47–48
fetal effects and, 92–93
future trends in, 105
gastrointestinal tract and, 39–40
history of, 10–13
immune system and, 48
labeling of, 24–25
laboratory testing and, 23
lipids and, 52–54
male reactions to women's use of, 218–19
means of action of, 17–18
menstrual irregularities and, 51
minerals and, 47
missed pills, 27–28
musculoskeletal system and, 46
myths about, 93–94
noncontraceptive health benefits of, 29–35
nose and, 48
over-the-counter use of, 18–19
pharmacology of, 13–15
physical examinations and, 22–23
pill switching, 28
reproductive tract and, 35–38
reproductive tract infections and, 48–51
resting and, 94
return of fertility and, 91–92
skin and, 43–46
smoking and, 62, 64–65
starting, 26–27
throat and, 48
types of, 15–17
urinary tract and, 46–47
usage of, 25–26
use of, at perimenopause, 28–29

vitamins and, 47
weight and, 51
Ortho-Gynol, 234
Ortho (pharmaceutical company),
13
Osteoporosis
injectable contraceptives and,
129–30
prevention, 34–35, 84
Ovarian cancer, 30–31, 84
Ovarian cysts, 31
Ovaries, oral contraceptives on, 38

Pain relief, 84
ParaGard intrauterine device, 140,
160, 161
Patches, contraceptive, 198–99
Patient-doctor relationships, 235–37
Pelvic inflammatory disease (PID),
50–51, 84
intrauterine devices and, 153–55
Perimenopause, use of oral
contraceptives at, 28–29
Periodic abstinence, 184–85
advantages of, 190
Billings method for, 187–88
calendar method for, 186
cervical mucus method for,
187–88
congenital abnormalities and,
188–89
disadvantages of, 190–91
effectiveness of, 189–90
lactating women and, 195–96
symptothermal method for, 188
temperature method for, 187–88
Pessaries, 4
Phasic pills, 16–17
Physical examinations,
contraceptives and, 22–23
Pill, the. *See* Oral contraceptives
Pincus, Gregory Goodwin, 11, 12,
13
Pituitary glands, oral contraceptives
and, 41
Pituitary microadenomas, 85
Placenta, folklore about, 3
Plan B, 103

Planned Parenthood Federation of
America, 11
Pliny the Elder, 8
Polycystic ovarian disease, 85
Polypoid hyperplasia, 36
Pomeroy method of sterilization,
200
POPs (progestin-only pills), 97–99
Population Council, 138
Porphyria, 85
Postabortion/postpartum, 85
Potencies, of oral contraceptives, 15
Pregnancies, 86. *See also*
Contraception
folklore about, 2
methods for preventing
unwanted, 3–4
role of gender and, 2
spacing of, 192–93
Premenstrual syndrome (PMS), 86
Prentif Cavity Rim Cervical Cap,
176
PREVEN, 102, 103
Progestasert intrauterine device,
160, 161
Progesterone, 10–11
Progesterone-T intrauterine devices,
140–41
Progestin-only pills (POPs), 97–99
Progestins, 11
for male contraception, 217
in oral contraceptives, 14–15

Queen Anne's lace, 7

Reality Female Condom, 182
Reproductive tract infections, oral
contraceptives and, 48–51
Research and development. *See*
Contraceptive research and
development
Resting, oral contraceptives and, 94
Rheumatoid arthritis, 34, 86
Rhythm. *See* Periodic abstinence
Rice-Wray, Edris, 13
Richter, Richard, 137
Robins, A. H., 141
Rock, John, 12

Roosevelt, Eleanor, 12
RU 486, 232–33

Sanger, Margaret, 11–12
Schistosomiasis, 86
Seizures, oral contraceptives and,
    86–87
Sequential pills, 16
Sexually transmitted diseases
    (STDs), 36, 87
    barrier contraceptives and, 167
    contraceptive implants and,
        113–14
Sheaths. *See* Condoms, male
Shug, 214
Sickle cell disease, 87
Silphium plant, 7
Skin conditions, oral contraceptives
    and, 43–46
SLE (systemic lupus eruthematosus),
    89
Smoking, 87–88
    oral contraceptives and, 62,
        64–65
Sperm, 187
    in preejaculatory fluid, 208–9
    scientific study of, 205–6
Spermicides, 168–69
    advantages of, 171
    disadvantages of, 171
    effectiveness of, 169
    safety of, 169–70
    using, 169
Sponges, contraceptive, 178–82
STDs. *See* Sexually transmitted
    diseases (STDs)
Sterilization
    ancient methods of, 8
    female, 199–203
    male, 213–15
    pregnancy rates following, 201–3
Sterlys intrauterine devices, 140
Steroids, 88
Stone, Abraham, 208
Storks, 2
Strokes, 88
    risk of, 62–63

Subdermal implants. *See* Implants,
    contraceptive
Sunday start, 26–27
Surgery, 88
Syntex Corporation, 10–11
Systemic lupus erythematosus
    (SLE), 89

Tatum, Howard, 139
Tatum-T intrauterine devices, 139,
    161
TCu 380 Ag intrauterine devices,
    140
TCu-380A intrauterine devices, 140
TCu 220C intrauterine devices, 140
Temperature method, for periodic
    abstinence, 187–88
Tension headaches, clinical
    management of, 71–72
Thalassemia, 89
Throat, oral contraceptives and, 48
Thromboembolism, risk of, 60–62
Thrombophlebitis, 89
Throphoblastic disease, 89
Thyroid disease, 89
Thyroid glands, oral contraceptives
    and, 41
Tietze, Christopher, 138
Toxic shock syndrome (TSS), 34
Triglycerides, 52
Triphasic oral contraceptives, 105
TSS (toxic shock syndrome), 34
Tubal disease, 32
Tuberculosis (TB), 89
Tyler, Edward T., 13

Uchida method of sterilization, 200
Ulcerative colitis, 89–90
United States
    contraceptive research and
        development in, 222–25
    litigious climate in, 242
    loss of leadership role in
        contraceptive research and
        development by, 237
    over-the-counter pill use in,
        18–19

Unwanted pregnancies, approaches
for preventing, 6–7. *See also*
Emergency contraceptives
Urinary tract, oral contraceptives
and, 46–47
Urinary tract infections, 90
Uterine fibroids, 33–34, 90
Uterus
ancient Egyptian beliefs about, 3
ancient Greek beliefs about, 3
oral contraceptives and, 37–38

Vaccines, contraceptive, 204
Vagina, oral contraceptives and,
36
Vaginal bleeding, 90, 126–27
Vaginal contraceptive sponges,
178–80
advantages of, 182
disadvantages of, 182
effectiveness of, 180
safety of, 181–82
using, 180
Vaginal rings, 197–98

Varicose veins, oral contraceptives
and, 46, 90–91
Vasectomies, 213–15
Vimule caps, 175
Vitamins, oral contraceptives and,
47
Vomiting, clinical management of,
70

Weight gain, oral contraceptives
and, 51, 91
WHO (World Health
Organization), 74
Withdrawal, 206–9
Worcester Foundation for
Experimental Biology, 11, 12
World Health Organization
(WHO), 74
Wyeth Laboratories, 13

Yasmin, 105
Yuzpe method, 100–101

Zipper, Jaime, 139